Contents

About Exit International

Founded in 1996 by Dr Philip Nitschke, Exit International (non-profit) is a global leader in the provision of end of life information to Seniors, people suffering serious illness & their families.

At the heart of Exit International's activities are Exit Workshops which are held regularly in Nth America, the UK, Ireland, New Zealand & Australia. Exit also runs an active & highly productive laboratory program.

Exit International USA is located in Bellingham (WA). Exit International is located in Australia. Exit operates chapters in towns & cities around the world.

For more information about Exit International, please visit:

http://www.exitinternational.net
http://www.peacefulpill.com

or email: *contact@exitinternational.net*

Phone: +1 360-347-1810 (USA)
+44 (0)20 7193 1557 (UK)
1300 10 3948 (EXIT) (within Australia)
+61 407-189-339 (outside Austrlia)

Content Revised:
September 2013

The Peaceful Pill Handbook

Dr Philip Nitschke

with

Dr Fiona Stewart

EXIT INTERNATIONAL USA

Published by Exit International USA
PO Box 4250
Bellingham WA 98227
USA

contact@exitinternational.net
Ph (+1) 360-347-1810

First published by Exit International US Ltd, 2006
Cover design by Branden Barber, Twin Lizards

The Peaceful Pill eHandbook
First published by Exit International US Ltd, 2008
Printed by Imprint Digital UK

Nitschke, Philip Haig.
        The peaceful pill handbook.

ISBN 978-0-9788788-7-0
www.peacefulpill.com
www.exitinternational.net

What the Critics said about

Killing Me Softly:
Voluntary Euthanasia & the Road to the Peaceful Pill
Dr Philip Nitschke & Dr Fiona Stewart

"The publication of this book will probably prove to be a landmark in the history of the reform of the unenlightened laws that restrict Australians' end-of-life choices." *Canberra Times*

"A fascinating book about a curly issue … it's a compelling, moving and important book about a difficult subject." *Sunday Mail*

"His passion screams from every page of this book … An informative read." *Launceston Examiner*

"For doctors especially, allow me to thoroughly recommend this book. The authors deliver a potent exposition of the role of medicine in this debate." *Australian Doctor*

"Killing Me Softly does represent, in a full and clear way, the issues surrounding voluntary euthanasia. To read it is to be better informed in the matter." *The West Australian*

"You'll either be for or against euthanasia but this book puts Nitschke and the debate in perspective." *Herald Sun*

"A fine new book" *The Mercury*

"Nitschke has never been shy about speaking out against the establishment and was already no friend of the medical one." *The Big Issue*

Disclaimer

While every effort has been exercised to avoid errors in the information contained in this book, neither the authors nor the publisher warrants that the information is error or omission free.

The Peaceful Pill Forums

Members of Exit International have free access (on approval) to the *Peaceful Pill* Discussion Forums at peacefulpillforums.com

This is an online space where members can ask questions about issues covered in the *eHandbook*, & benefit from the comments, advice and experience of experts, other subscribers and Exit members.

To join the Forums, click the link and register.

www.peacefulpillforums.com

Preface

The Peaceful Pill Handbook addresses an important need amongst at Seniors and those who are seriously ill about how to access the best information about end-of-life choices.

In 1996, Australia passed the world's first right to die law; the *Rights of the Terminally Ill Act (ROTI)*. Under *ROTI*, four of my seriously ill patients self-administered a legal, lethal overdose of drugs; a Peaceful Pill if you like. All died peacefully in their sleep, surrounded by people they loved.

I know this, because back then I was their treating physician. I was the one who put the needle into their veins. And I was the one who built the 'Deliverance Machine' that they used to die. The Deliverance Machine was a laptop computer and program that gave these individuals the ultimate control over their deaths. Their deaths taught me much, but mostly how important it is for peole to be allowed to have control at the end.

On each separate occasion, the computer presented a short series of questions:

1. Are you aware that if you go ahead to the last screen and press the 'yes' button you will be given a lethal dose of medications and die?
2. Are you certain you understand that if you proceed and press the 'yes' button on the next screen you will die?
3. In 15 seconds you will be given a lethal injection … press 'yes' to proceed.

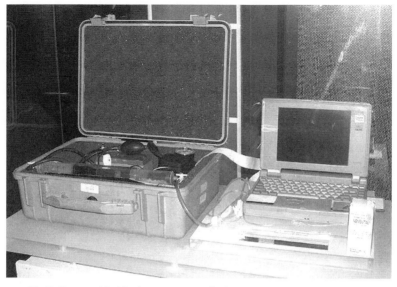

The Deliverance Machine is on permanent display at the British Science Museum

After pressing the button for a third time, the Machine would deliver a lethal dose of the barbiturate, Nembutal. The Deliverance Machine enabled these four people to die peacefully and with dignity under a new law.

My experience in those days of legal, assisted suicide taught me that the drug sodium pentobarbital - commonly known as Nembutal - provides one of the most peaceful death imaginable. And it almost never fails. That is why it is used in countries like the Netherlands, Belgium and Switzerland and the US States of Oregon, Washington, Montana & Vermont where assisted suicide is lawful.

In countries like Australia, Canada, the UK and the remaining American states, where there are no end-of-life laws, the means of achieving a peaceful death is next to impossible. In Australia - my birthplace - for the past decade the Government has made it increasingly difficult for Seniors and people who are seriously ill to access information about their end-of-life choices. The Australian Government seems more concerned to keep people in the dark. Their rationale is that if people are kept in a state of complete ignorance they will live longer, happier lives. NOT True!

In my experience, once people have access to information that empowers and enables informed decisions to be made, they tend to stop worrying. Knowing one's options enables a person to make considered decisions as a matter of course. Knowledge about one's end-of-life choices is empowering. It is this empowerment that promotes a longer, happier life. NOT Ignorance.

Preface

Acknowledgements

The Peaceful Pill eHandbook could not have been written without the support of many people. First to thank are the many Exit members who have contributed their expertise, ideas and travel stories. This is truly a joint effort.

Secondly, the staff at Exit International we thank very sincerely for all they do day in, day out. Outside of Exit, special thanks to Steve Hopes of iKandy Films in Sydney, Branden Barber in San Franciso and the technical staff at Yudu in the UK. Finally, we'd like to thank our publisher, Richard West.

Dr Philip Nitschke
Bellingham, Washington

A Word of Caution

This book *is* intended for Seniors and people who are seriously ill (and their families). This book is *not* intended for young people or anyone suffering from psychiatric illness or depression. As authors we acknowledge that there is a small risk that this book may be misused by people for whom this information is clearly not appropriate.

The risk that information of this nature may be misused was a fact acknowledged by the 'godfather' of the right-to-die movement, former British journalist, Derek Humphry. When Derek first published *Final Exit* in 1991 he was criticised for endangering suicidal teens the world over. However, as he would later point out, the suicide statistics have failed to show the much talked about 'blip'. There has been no rise in the suicide rate. Providing people with information does not incite or encourage people to die. And this is a critical point.

Rather, reliable, accurate information empowers people to make make informed decisions about their own end-of-life circumstances. Good information should not only prevent grim, horrible deaths of gunshot and hanging (the most common causes of suicide in the US, UK and Australia respectively) but it should allay fears. It is paradox, perhaps. By equipping Seniors and those who are seriously ill with knowledge that empowers and returns control, these same people are more likely to stop worrying and get on with living. Anecdotal evidence to this effect can be seen at each and every Exit meeting. Fears are addressed and participants feel back in control.

As principal author I ask that users of this Book respect its integrity and intended audience. Seniors and people who are seriously ill, deserve to be able to make informed decisions about their futures. Ignorance is not an acceptable state of affairs.

It is a basic human right to live and die with one's dignity in tact. *The Peaceful Pill Handbook* is one way of helping ensure that one's passing might be as proud and strong as one's living.

Note: Purchasers of the Print edition *Peaceful Pill Handbook* are entitled to a US$10 cashback should they choose to elect to upgrade to a subscription to the online *Peaceful Pill eHandbook*.

Once a reader upgrades by taking out a subscription at *www.peacefulpill.com*, email Exit with proof of purchase & we will credit $10 to you by check.

1

End of Life Considerations

Developing an End of Life Plan

People make end of life plans for all sorts of reasons. Some people are concerned that one day they will become so sick and frail and their quality of life will become so impaired that death will become the preferred option. Others worry that because current generations are living longer than their parents' and grandparents' generations, they will have to face that new set of worries that come from longevity itself. Some elderly people are simply 'tired of life.'

The reasons that lead an elderly person or someone who is seriously ill to seek information about their end-of-life choices are many and varied. All are intensely personal. Rewriting the ways in which society can plan for and experience death and dying is the challenge of our time.

The development of an end of life plan is one small step that all of us can take to protect those we love from the ravages of the law. While most of us will never use our plan, we can all draw comfort in knowing that if things ever become too painful or undignified (especially in the context of serious illness and age), we will have a plan in place that will allow us to maintain our dignity and our independence.

The Wonders of Modern Medicine

In any discussion of end of life issues the role of modern medicine is paramount. While no one can be critical of the huge advances in medical science over recent decades - improving beyond measure the length and quality of our lives – there is also a flip side. In contrast to previous generations, we are now far more likely to die of slower, debilitating conditions that are associated with old age and illness. Yet we are also more likely to be kept alive through an increasingly sophisticated array of medical technologies.

A longer life can be a wonderful thing, but should we be forced to live on, if we come to a point where we have simply had enough? Surely the act of balancing one's quality of life against the struggle of daily living in our later years or in illness, should be each individual to arbitrate.

Our Ageing Population

A century ago when life expectancy was approximately 25 years less than it is today, few people had the opportunity to reflect on how they might die. Then people were much more likely to die quickly with little warning. For example, one hundred years ago infectious disease was common. People considered themselves lucky if they were still alive in their mid 50s. The widespread introduction of public health measures such as sewerage, water reticulation, good housing, and of course the introduction of modern antibiotics have all played a part in greatly reducing the toll of infectious disease.

In modern times, those living in the developed west have a life expectancy of 75 to 80 years. Now in industrialised countries, we will be more likely to experience diseases and disabilities that were rare in earlier times. While old age is not in itself predictive of serious physical illness, the gradual deterioration of one's body with age leads to an almost inevitable decline in a person's quality of life.

This is why we see the issue of control in dying as being an increasingly common concern for many elderly people. Exit's workshop program is often booked out months ahead as elderly folk seek answers to their practical questions about their end of life options. Although few who attend these workshops have any intention of dying in the near future, most see a need to organise and plan for this inevitable event.

Just as many of us plan for other aspects associated with dying (eg. we all write a will, appoint executors, and some of us prepay for funerals), so it is common sense to ensure that we have a plan about how we might wish to die. Yet to be in a position to plan for one's death, one must first know one's options. And that means information.

The Question of Suicide

Anyone who makes plans for their own death can be said to be planning their own suicide. While for some people suicide is a tainted concept, for a growing number of older people it is an issue of great interest and discussion. In this context, suicide is a way out of a life that an individual might consider is not worth living.

People who come to Exit workshops are well aware of the importance of making that ultimate of decisions, the decision to die. They are all acutely aware of the need to get it right. In this Chapter, we examine the phenomenon of suicide in the context of the modern life course, and why access to the best in end of life information is so important.

A Brief History of Suicide

Over the years, the way in which society views the taking of one's own life has varied enormously. Suicide has not always been seen as the act of a sick and depressed person. In ancient Greece, Athenian magistrates kept a supply of poison for anyone who wanted to die. You just needed official permission. For the Stoics of ancient times, suicide was considered an appropriate response, if the problems of pain, grave illness or physical abnormalities became too great.

With the rise of Christianity, however, suicide came to be viewed as a sin (a violation of the sixth commandment). As Lisa Lieberman writes in her book *Leaving You*, all of a sudden 'the Roman ideal of heroic individualism' was replaced 'with a platonic concept of submission to divine authority'.

It was Christianity that changed society's view of suicide from the act of a responsible person, to an infringement upon the rights of God. One's death became a matter of God's will, not one's own and it was at this point that penalties were first established for those who attempted suicide. If the suicide was successful, it was the family of the offender who were punished with fines and social disgrace.

With the emergence of modern medicine in the 19th Century, the meaning of suicide changed again and it is this understanding that prevails today. Suicide is now generally thought of as an illness. If a person wants to end their life, then they must be sick (psychiatric illness, with depression the usual diagnosis). The appropriate response, therefore, is medical treatment (in the form of psychiatric counselling and/or anti-depressant medications).

At Exit International, we question the view of suicide that automatically links a person's decision to die to depression and mental illness. Are we seriously postulating that the suicide bombers of the Middle East are depressed? Rather, the act of suicide must be seen as context dependent.

For example, a person who is very elderly and who is seeing friends die around them on a weekly basis and who must be wondering 'am I next?' is going to have a very different outlook on dying than the young person who has their whole life in front of them. Likewise, when serious illness is present. A person's attitude towards death must be understood in the context of that person's situation.

In Oregon, where physician-assisted suicide (PAS) is legal, symptoms of depression have been found in 20 per cent of patients who request PAS (Battle, 2003). A 1998 study by the

Australian Bureau of Statistics reported 15 per cent of men and 18 per cent of women who suicided had 'an associated or contributory diagnosis of a mental disorder' (ABS, 2000). At Exit we argue that feelings of sadness (as opposed to clinical depression) are a normal response to a diagnosis of a serious illness.

This is why some studies continue to find a sadness associated with a serious illness. You don't need to be a psychiatrist to understand that this might be a normal response to an extraordinary situation (Ryan, 1996). To assume that suicide amongst the elderly or people who are seriously ill is the result of depression or other psychiatric illness, is to adopt uncritically a biomedical way of seeing the world. We can do better.

Suicide & Depression

The link between suicide and depression remains a vexed issue with millions of dollars in government funding devoted to raising the community's awareness of suicide, especially amongst the young and some minority groups (eg. farmers). And there can be no doubt. People who suffer from clinical depression are clearly at risk of suicide. Severe depressive states can rob a person of the ability to make rational decisions and these people need care and treatment until they are once again able to resume control. Yet illness of this severity is not common and needs to be distinguished from a larger group of people who show occasional signs of depression but who are in full control of their actions.

There is a significant difference between a person having moments of feeling down or having a transitory feeling that their life has lost purpose and the person who has severe clinical depression, where even the most basic daily decisions of life become problematic.

This is quite different from an elderly or seriously ill person's desire to formulate an end of life plan; a plan whose sole aim is to maintain control over their final days. People who like to be prepared and who are not depressed should not be viewed in psychiatric terms.

End of Life Decisions & the Role of Palliative Care

Critics of Voluntary Euthanasia and Assisted Suicide often argue that if palliative care is available and of good enough standard, patients will never need ask for assistance to die. This is untrue, but to understand the claim, one needs to look at the background of the palliative care speciality.

Palliative care was the first branch of medicine to shift the focus away from 'cure at all costs' and to focus instead upon the treatment and management of symptoms (for people who have a life-threatening illness). In this sense, palliative care's aim has never been 'cure'. Rather, palliative medicine is about symptom control. It is about improving the quality of life of those who are seriously ill and dying.

To date, palliative care has been most successful in the treatment of pain. Indeed, it is often claimed - perhaps exaggeratedly - that palliative care can successfully address pain in 95 per cent of all cases. What is much less spoken about is the speciality's limited ability to alleviate some other common symptoms of serious disease; symptoms such as weakness, breathlessness or nausea. Or, quite simply to guarantee a good death.

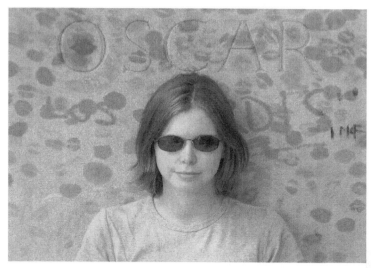

Angelique Flowers at Oscar Wilde's grave at Pere Lachaise cemetery in Paris in 2006.

No where can the shortcomings of palliative care be more obvious than in the tragic death in August 2008 of 31 year old Melbourne writer, Angelique Flowers. At the age of 15 years, Angelique was diagnosed with painful Crohn's Disease. On 9 May 2008, shortly before her 31st birthday she was diagnosed with Stage 4 colon cancer.

As Angelique said, in one of the several videos she made in the weeks leading up to her death, there is no Stage 5. At Stage 4 and upon diagnosis, the cancer had already spread to her liver and ovaries. Angie's doctors told her then, her days were numbered. They also told her that there would be very little they could do to ensure that her death was pain-free and dignified.

As history now tells Angelique's story, this courageous, clever, beautiful young woman died in the most difficult and unpleasant way. As a patient in Australia's premiere palliative care unit at Monash Medical Centre in Melbourne, Angelique's care was the best that modern medicine can provide, and that money can buy. Despite some hiccups, Angelique's pain control was described as reasonable. What was not so good and what the law prevents medicine from addressing, was her death.

Angelique Flowers died vomiting up faecal matter after experiencing an acute bowel blockage. Just as her doctors had warned, her death was simply awful. They had told her that it could be shocking, and it was.

This young woman was terrified of this possibility which is why she put out a call for Nembutal, on the Internet. Although Angie was successful at obtaining Nembutal, because of the law she kept the drug hidden at her parents' home. When the bowel blockage occurred, Angelique was in the hospice yet her Nembutal was at home. She lost her chance to take control.

Shortly before she died, Angie made a video diary. In it she pleaded with Australian Prime Minister Kevin Rudd to once again, legalise voluntary euthanasia in Australia. Angelique's tragic story shows many things, including why a modern, civilised society needs the best palliative care and voluntary euthanasia/ assisted suicide.

At Exit, we are frequently approached by people who tell us that their palliative care is second to none but who, like Angelique, still wish to be in control of their death. They say that while they might not now be in pain, the quality of their life is nonetheless seriously effected by their illness. They know that there is often nothing that modern palliative medicine can do about it.

Some of these people are so weak that they cannot move unassisted. Others have shortness of breath which makes independent living impossible. For a significant number of people, it is non-medical issues that have most impact upon the quality of their life.

One recent memorable case concerned a middle aged man called Bob. Bob was suffering from lung cancer. He was incredibly sad that his favourite past time - a round of gold with his mates - was no longer possible. This person was clear. It was his frustration at being house-bound and dependent on visits from friends and family, rather than the physical symptoms of the cancer, that made him choose an elective death.

Palliative care is no universal panacea. While this branch of medicine does have a valuable contribution to make, especially in the field of pain control, it is unhelpful to use symptom management as the benchmark against which a person's quality of life is measured.

Rather, people rate their quality of life in different ways with no two individuals' assessment the same. While a life without pain is clearly better than a life with pain, this is not always the most important issue. Instead it is that person's own complex assessment of their life's worth that is the key. The physical symptoms of an illness are often only one of many considerations. Just ask Angelique.

The Tired of Life Phenomenon

In recent years, a new trend has begun to emerge; one that has caused Exit to rethink our approach to death and dying. Increasingly at our workshops, we meet elderly people who are fit and healthy (for their age), but for whom life has become increasingly burdensome. Such people are not depressed. Rather, the sentiment expressed is that 'I have lived enough of the good life and now it's time to go.' The actions of Australian couple, Sidney and Marjorie Croft, explain this phenomenon well.

In 2002, the Crofts sent Exit International their suicide note explaining why they had decided to go together. Exit had no prior knowledge of the couple's plans. We knew only that they had attended several Exit workshops where they sat at the back, holding hands and asking questions.

The Crofts did not need to write this note yet they wanted us to understand. And in return they asked for our respect.

To Whom it May Concern

Please don't condemn us, or feel badly of us for what we have done.

We have thought clearly of this for a long time and it has taken a long time to get the drugs needed.

We are in our late 80s and 90 is on the horizon. At this stage, would it be wrong to expect no deterioration in our health? More importantly, would our mental state be bright and alert?

In 1974 we both lost our partners whom we loved very dearly. For two and a half years Marjorie became a recluse with her grief, and Sid became an alcoholic. We would not like to go through that traumatic experience again. Hence we decided we wanted to go together.

We have no children and no one to consider.

We have left instructions that we be cremated and that our ashes be mixed together. We feel that way, we will be together forever.

Please don't feel sad, or grieve for us. But feel glad in your heart as we do.

Sidney and Marjorie Croft

The Crofts are the private face of an increasingly common sentiment among a minority of older people; that is that a good life should be able to be brought to an end with a good death, when and if a person so wishes. To suggest, as many in the medical profession have done, that the Crofts were 'depressed' is to trivialise and patronise them for their actions.

Another person who evoked this 'tired of life' phenomenon was retired French academic, Lisette Nigot. In 2002, Lisette Nigot also took her own life, consuming lethal drugs she had stockpiled over the years. Lisette's reason for dying? She said she did not want to turn 80.

Lisette Nigot insisted that she had led a good and full life. She said she had always known that she would not want to become 'too old.' 'I do not take to old age very well' she told film-maker Janine Hosking whose feature documentary *Mademoiselle and the Doctor* traced the last months of her life.

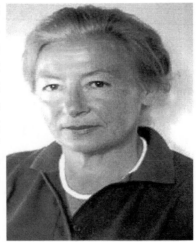

Mademoiselle Lisette Nigot

In late 2002, shortly before her 80th birthday, Lisette Nigot ended her life. Intelligent and lucid to the end, Lisette knew her own mind. A fiercely independent woman, it is not surprising that she expected control in her dying, just as she had in her own life. In *Mademoiselle and the Doctor* she explained:

> 'I don't like the deterioration of my body ... I don't like not being able to do the things I used to be able to do ... and I don't like the discrepancy there is between the mind which remains what it always was, and the body which is sort of physically deteriorating.
>
> Perhaps my mind will go and I would hate that. And certainly my body will go and I wouldn't be very happy with that either. So I might as well go while the going is good'.

When details of the Croft's and Lisette Nigot's death were made public, many tried to medicalise their situations. An assortment of diseases and conditions were suggested as reasons for their decision to end their lives. Underpinning all of this was the belief that 'well' people do not take their own life.

Then Australian Prime Minister John Howard, commenting on Lisette Nigot's actions, stated, 'I have a strong belief that we should not be encouraging well people to take their own life, I'm appalled.'

At Exit we do not encourage anyone, sick or well, to take their own life. We do, however, believe that a decision to end one's life can be rational. Such a decision can occur just as much in the context of age as in the context of serious suffering and disease. This is why all elderly people should have access to reliable end of life information; information which is critical if mistakes are to be prevented.

Exit Workshops

In recent years, Exit's workshops have grown in popularity spreading over Australia, NZ, UK, USA and Canada. From their commencement in 1997, this flagship Exit program now provides factual, accurate information to over 4000 people every year.

The workshop idea was first coined in 1997 after the world's first end of life law - the *Rights of the Terminally Ill Act* - was overturned by the Australian parliament. At that time, the Voluntary Euthanasia Research Foundation - as Exit was then known - was approached by increasing numbers of older people who wanted to know their end of life options. These people were not ill. Rather, they wanted to know what their options were, should they ever become ill.

Unable to visit these rational, elderly adults on a one-on-one basis, Exit Director Philip Nitschke began workshops, initially with around 20 people at a time. Held in local community centres, the workshops provided a perfect opportunity to correct misinformation and answer questions.

Since that time workshops have only gotten bigger, now attracting over 100 participants at each meeting. Because Exit can still not keep up with people's desire to obtain end of life information, this book has been created. Welcome to Exit's new global workshop.

Conclusion

If one is to suggest that the elderly and seriously ill have the right - for good and sound reasons - to end their lives earlier than nature would have it, then the provision of accurate, up-to-date information is an important first step.

Information is the main reason why people join Exit International. Information is certainly the main reason why our workshops are booked out months ahead. People want to know how to end their lives peacefully, reliably and with dignity. Most people know that they may never use this information. All are comforted, however, in knowing that if things 'turn bad' as they put it, they have a plan in place.

Remember, suicide is legal, yet assisting a suicide is illegal. This is why everyone should develop an end of life plan. An end of life plan will keep one's family and loved ones safe from the law. An end of life plan is the responsible thing to do.

2

Voluntary Euthanasia, Suicide & the Law

In most western countries, suicide is legal, yet assisted suicide is a crime, attracting harsh legal penalties. While a person who takes their own life commits no crime, a person found guilty of assisting another can face a long jail term.

Think about it. The law makes it a crime for a person to assist another person to do something that is lawful. There is no other example of this in modern western legal systems. This is why any person who chooses to be involved in the death of another - however tangentially and for whatever reasons – needs to be very careful indeed. This is especially true when friends and family are involved and emotions may cloud one's judgement.

Legal Definitions & Penalties

Technically speaking Voluntary Euthanasia is the term used to describe the situation when a medical professional might administer to a patient a lethal injection. Voluntary euthanasia is legal in countries such as the Netherlands and Belgium.

By contrast, Physician Assisted Suicide (PAS) is the term that describes when a medical professional might prescribe, but not administer, a lethal drug to a patient. An example of this is the US states of Oregon, Washington, Montana and Vermont.

Finally, the term Assisted Suicide describes the situation in Switzerland where the provision of lethal drugs to people who are suffering has long been decriminalised.

Generally speaking, assisting a suicide is legally defined as 'advising,' 'counselling' or 'assisting' a person to end their life. Sometimes the words 'aid and abet' are also used. In most countries assisting a suicide carries severe legal penalties.

In Australia, the penalty ranges from 5 years to life imprisonment, depending upon the jurisdiction. In Britain (and Canada) the penalty extends to 14 years. In 2009, the UK director of public prosecutions, Keir Starmer, issued new guidelines on assisted suicide following a successful campaign by MS sufferer Debbie Purdy to seek clarification of the law. See:*http://www.cps.gov.uk/ news/press_releases/144_09/*

In the US, assisting a suicide is illegal in just over half of all states, with the remainder treating it the same as the crime of murder or manslaughter. In the US, the penalties for assisted suicide vary from state to state. The only exceptions are the states of Oregon, Washington, Montana and Vermont where Physician Assisted Suicide (PAS) is legal in some circumstances.

In Michigan, the late Dr Jack Kevorkian was incarcerated for almost a decade for the assisted suicide of his terminally ill patient, Thomas Youk. In March 1999, Kevorkian was convicted of second degree murder and sentenced to 10 to 25 years jail.

Defining Assisted Suicide

So what is assisted suicide? At the current time, argument about what actually constitutes 'assisted suicide' shows no sign of easing. A significant grey area continues to exist at the boundaries, with lawyers unable to give clear and concise answers to many questions about this issue.

The dearth of case law leaves it unclear about whether, for example, giving a person the information they need, or even sitting with a person while they take their own life, is assisting with their suicide. On the one hand there is the argument that the mere act of sitting with someone about to suicide provides psychological encouragement? Or does it? Perhaps those present have a duty of care to prevent that person from harming themselves? Perhaps one should leap from one's chair and grab the glass of lethal drugs from the person's lips? But wouldn't that be an assault? The law regarding assisted suicide is ill defined and murky.

VE Legislation - What Type of Law is Needed?

Over the years, legislation has attempted to bring clarity and order to the Assisted Suicide debate. By defining the class of person who can be helped to die and by stipulating the manner in which this help can be provided, laws such as the *Rights of the Terminally Ill Act (Northern Territory)* - the world's first right-to-die law - went a long way towards establishing uniformity and equity.

To make use of the law a person had to be 'terminally ill,' and this was defined in the Act. The person also had to satisfy a number of other strict criteria.

If they qualified, they obtained the right to request lawful assistance from a doctor to die. Other laws (Oregon, Holland etc) have also set out to define exactly which group of people can have help to die. In all cases, eligibility is tightly controlled.

Yet even where VE laws work well, there is one significant drawback. The very strict set of conditions means that the process of establishing eligibility is demanding and can be humiliating to those involved.

Besides, there are some people (those who fit the 'tired of life' description) who will simply never qualify. In the Northern Territory, a terminally ill person had to obtain two medical opinions, a palliative care review and a psychiatric consultation before they could qualify to use the law to die. In practice, this meant that some very sick people had to beg the medical profession in order to qualify to die.

In the course of my involvement with this law, it quickly became apparent that none of my four patients who used the *ROTI Act* would have bothered with the exhaustive assessment process if they had access to a Peaceful Pill at home in the cupboard. Why would a person subject themselves to a compulsory psychiatric examination, if they already had the means to a peaceful, dignified death?

They would simply have waited till the time was right and then taken the Pill. The very laws that were supposed to empower these sick and frail people seemed to do the exact opposite. The law denied these individuals' control. Instead, control was placed in the hands of those doctors tasked with establishing eligibility.

While some people may wish to involve doctors in their deaths, others do not. Our point at Exit is that death need not be a medical event. It is also arguable whether the medical profession should be given the role of arbiter, of who gets the right to die with dignity, and who does not.

(An extensive discussion of Exit's philosophy of death and dying can be found in *Killing Me Softly: VE and the Road to the Peaceful Pill*, Penguin, 2005 - republshed in 2011 by Exit US and available from Exit). This medical model of death and dying hangs over us and needs to be challenged. This is, in part, why this book has been produced. The Internet Age has proven perfect for the democratisation of information.

Conclusion

There are many understandable reasons why a seriously ill person (or an elderly person) should be encouraged to make an end of life plan. Exit does not accept the proposition that seriously ill people who plan for the end of their life are either depressed or mentally ill.

Rather, a person's right to end-of-life information is better understood as critical to empowering that person to make their own considered decisions and choices, just as they have done all their life.

By implementing laws that restrict and withhold this information, the State is behaving in a way that is not only cruel, but inequitable and unjust. Those with money and connections will always be better resourced, better able to get the necessary information and better able to access the restricted drugs, than those who are less well off. This book is intended to restore the balance.

3

What is a Peaceful Pill?

Introduction

The Peaceful Pill is a pill or drink that provides a peaceful, pain-free death at a time of a person's individual choosing; a pill that is orally ingested and available to 'most' people.

Dr Philip Nitschke

It was the late Dutch Supreme Court Judge Huib Drion who first called for the introduction of a Pill. In a letter to the editor of the Dutch newspaper *NRC/Handelsblad*, Drion openly bemoaned the fact that while his doctor friends knew what to do and how to access the right drugs for a peaceful death, as a lawyer he did not.

Drion questioned the logic of why he, a retired judge, should not have the same ready access to a dignified death as his doctor friends. According to Drion, all people over a certain age should have the right to die at a time of their choosing. A pill, he argued, would confer this right.

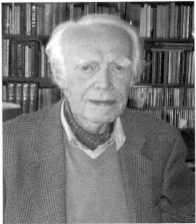

Fig 3.1: Professor Huib Drion

Elderly and ailing people often realize that, at some time in the future, they could well find themselves in an unacceptable and unbearable situation, one that is worsening. A pill to end life at one's own discretion could alleviate some of their anxiety. Not a pill for now, but for the unforeseeable future so that the end can be humane (Huib Drion, Dikkers cited in Nitschke and Stewart, 2005)

Following Drion, Exit research has confirmed that a Peaceful Pill provides peace of mind for its seriously ill or elderly owner, giving that person a sense of control over their life and death. Unlike end of life laws that depend solely upon a person's state of health (or illness), Drion's 'universal model' has only one criteria, that of age.

Drion suggested that *all* people over the age of 65 years should have access to a Pill. While the age is arguable, the point remains the same. The 'Drion Pill' or 'Peaceful Pill' should be accessible to the seriously ill *as well as* the elderly.

The History of the Suicide Pill

The idea of a Peaceful Pill – that is, a lethal substance or liquid that can be orally ingested – is not new. In Athenian times, the herb Hemlock was the drug of choice for suicide and it was taken as a drink. The most famous Hemlock suicide was that of the Greek critical scholar, Socrates.

In more modern times, the chemical compound Cyanide has been widely employed as a suicide pill. One recent well known death from Cyanide was that of Spanish quadriplegic Ramon Sampedro.

In 1998, Sampedro ended his life by drinking cyanide that had been provided and prepared by his friends. The award-winning 2004 film *The Sea Inside* provides a remarkable account of his life and death.

For much of the 20th Century, cyanide was routinely issued to intelligence agents as part of their job. Hitler's head man in the SS and the Gestapo, Heinrich Himmler, escaped interrogation upon arrest by the British, by swallowing a capsule of cyanide.

Hermann Goering, head of the Luftwaffe, avoided the hangman by taking potassium cyanide the night before the planned execution. Where the purpose is to avoid interrogation and torture, speed of action is essential and cyanide fitted the bill.

The Best Peaceful Pill

Fifty years on and it is pentobarbital (Nembutal) that is favoured as an ideal Peaceful Pill. Nembutal is a member of the barbiturate family of drugs that are made from the salts of barbituric acid. These active barbiturate salts have been used medically for many years, mainly as sedatives or sleeping tablets.

In the 1950s, for example, there were more than 20 marketed forms of barbiturate sleeping tablets. Early examples included Veronal, Amytal, Seconal, Soneryl, and, of course, Nembutal. Fifty years ago, Nembutal was a widely prescribed drug, recommended even to help babies sleep, and to calm aching teeth (See Fig 13.1)

Over the last 30 years the barbiturates have slowly disappeared from the market. The fact that in overdose they caused death, either accidentally or deliberately, and the availability of newer, safer sleeping drugs has led to their decline. Nembutal was removed from the Australian prescribing schedule in 1998. The last barbiturate sleeping tablet, Amytal, was removed in 2003.

Perceived Benefits of a Peaceful Pill

There are many means by which a seriously ill person can end their life, although relatively few of these methods are reliable, dignified and peaceful. In most western countries, hanging and gun shot remain the most common methods of suicide.

Yet few people would resort to such means if they had any real choice. Most seriously ill or elderly people who are considering death, seek a method that is peaceful, dignified and pain free. Commonly this is expressed as, 'I simply want to go to sleep and die'

In 2004, Exit International undertook a major study of our supporters' attitudes to various methods of dignified dying (n=1163).

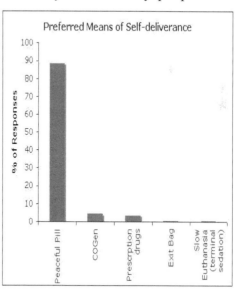

Fig 3.2: Survey of Exit Members
Methods of Self Deliverance

What we found was a strong and significant preference for a Pill over all other methods. Indeed, 89% of respondents (average age 72 years) said that they would prefer to take a Pill than use a plastic Exit bag, a carbon monoxide generator (COGenie) or seek help from a doctor to provide them with 'slow euthanasia.' A 'Pill' was defined as something that could be taken as a single oral dose (by mouth) in either tablet form or as a small drink.

The reasons behind the respondents' preferences became clear as more of the data set was examined. Most of those surveyed saw the Peaceful Pill as an important way of providing independence (91%). It was seen as an advantage if one did not have to depend on friends and family for assistance when the time came.

A Peaceful Pill was also seen to provide 'peace of mind' (90%), was reliable (88%) and, unlike the Exit Bag or the Carbon Monoxide Generator, the Pill was easy-to-administer (87%) since it required no equipment and no technical know-how.

In this way, the Peaceful Pill was seen as a method that was accessible and usable, even by the most frail.

Conclusion

Exit's survey has established a strong preference for a reliable and effective Peaceful Pill as the best means of providing the option of a peaceful death at the time of one's choosing. Much of the remainder of this book focuses on the various forms a Peaceful Pill might take.

In providing this information we are following the agenda set by long-standing members of Exit International.

4

The Exit RP Test

Many end of life options are discussed in this book and it can be a daunting project trying to distinguish or compare the relative advantages or shortcomings of one over the other. To simplify the process, we have developed a simple rating system that can be applied to all end of life methods. We call this the Reliability & Peacefulness Test – the 'Exit RP Test'.

Primary Criteria

The 'Exit RP Test' provides a benchmark against which all end of life options can be considered. The values addressed by the test came to Exit's attention through specific research on the notion of a Peaceful Pill and also through personal accounts and anecdotes over the past decade. This feedback continues to identify two principal factors in people's preferences for end of life methods. These factors are 'Reliability' and 'Peacefulness.'

In the RP Test, Reliability and Peacefulness are each given a score of 1 to 10. The higher the number, the more reliable and peaceful the method in question. For example, Nembutal achieves a high overall score, hanging a very low score.

Reliability (R - 10)

Reliability has been consistently identified as a major important factor in assessing end of life methods. A seriously ill person wanting to end their life needs to know the method *will* work. No one wants to take chances with a method that *might* work. Reliability is essential.

Peacefulness (P - 10)

Peacefulness is the second major criteria identified by Exit. There is almost no interest in methods that are violent, irrespective of how reliable they might be.

The most commonly expressed wish by seriously ill and elderly people is that they be able to die in their sleep.

Secondary Criteria

There are a number of lesser, but nevertheless highly-desired, characteristics for a method of dying. Six additional secondary factors are listed below:

Availability (A)
Preparation and Administration (Pr)
Undetectability (U)
Speed of Effect (Sp)
Safety to Others (Sa)
Storage - Shelf Life (St)

In the RP test, a score of 1-5 is given for each of these secondary characteristics.

Availability (A - 5)

To be of any use the method must be available. The most peaceful and reliable drug is of no use if it is unavailable.

Preparation and Administration (Pr - 5)

Simplicity of preparation and administration is an important factor. No one wants to use complicated equipment that is difficult to assemble or drugs that are hard to use.

Undetectability (U - 5)

Methods that leave no obvious trace are strongly preferred. In reality, this might mean that an attending physician will be more likely to assume that the death has been caused by a known underlying disease. In this situation, the question of suicide does not arise.

Speed of Effect (Sp - 5)

Speed of death is a further significant factor. Speed limits the likelihood of discovery and any possible interference (resuscitation).

Safety to Others (Sa - 5)

Most seriously ill people do not want to die alone. Methods that present a danger to others are unpopular for this reason.

Storage - Shelf life (St - 5)

There is a strong preference for methods that use substances, drugs or items that do not deteriorate with time. This means the person should be able to assemble the required items or obtain the required drugs in advance, and not have to worry about linking the possible timing of one's passing to the acquisition of the items. All of the methods described in this book have been given an Exit RP Test score. The maximum possible is 50 points, the higher the score the 'better' the method. Some criteria will vary of course depending on an individual's particular circumstances. *The RP Test rating should only ever be used as a general guide.*

Take the example of the Exit Bag when used in conjunction with Helium (see Chapter 5).

Test Factor	**Score**
Reliability: This is good, but technique is important	R=8/10
Peacefulness: There is some short term awareness and alarm	P=7/10
Availability: Necessary items are readily available	A=5/5
Preparation: Items require assembly and coordination	Pr=1/5
Undetectability: If items removed, totally undetectable, even in the event of an autopsy	U=5/5
Speed: Unconsciousness and death occur quickly	Sp=5/5
Safety: The method presents no risk to others present	Sa=5/5

Storage:
Equipment does not deteriorate and testing   St=5/5 is
readily available

Total for Helium and an Exit Bag   41 (82%)

Now compare the RP Test result for the Exit Bag + Helium with
the Use of Sodium Cyanide (see Chapter 7).

Test Factor	Score
Reliability: This is very high	R=10/10
Peacefulness: Patchy reports, hard to assess	P=5/10
Availability: Difficult to obtain or manufacture	A=2/5
Preparation: This is straightforward	Pr=5/5
Undetectability: Some clinical changes may be noted, certainly noted on autopsy	U=3/5
Speed: Produces a rapid death	Sp=5/5
Safety: There may be some slight risk to those present from possible HCN gas production	Sa=3/5
Storage: Well packaged, shelf life indefinite	St=5/5

Total for Sodium Cyanide   38 (76%)

A Note of Caution

The RP Test score serves only as a guide. Individual circumstances and preferences will always influence a person's decision. There are people for whom a plastic Exit bag over their head will never be a viable option, no matter how peaceful and reliable the method.

This may be because of an individual's particular aesthetic concern and have nothing to do with the method's high reliability physiologically. Nevertheless, *if* this is a real concern, the method will not be considered, irrespective of the high RP Test score.

Similarly, the 'availability' of a particular method can differ from individual to individual. The comparison above suggests that helium would be preferred above cyanide.

However, if an individual has recently become so disabled through illness that the use of an Exit Bag is physically impossible, and yet that same person has access to cyanide powder, the final choice will clearly not be determined by the highest RP Test score.

See Table 1 which provides the overall RP Test scores for the six approaches described in this book.

5

Hypoxic Death & the Exit Bag

Introduction

The plastic Exit Bag provides people with the means to obtain a simple, effective and peaceful death. While Exit research has found that relatively few people would *prefer* to use a Plastic Bag over the simple ingestion of a Peaceful Pill, it remains one of the most accessible methods available.

There is much misinformation, however, about how a plastic Exit Bag works and why it is so effective. The common assumption is that the bag causes death by 'suffocation'.

Suffocation occurs when a person cannot easily take a breath. Examples of this include tying a rope around the neck, or pushing a pillow into one's face. The act of mechanically blocking one's breathing is *terrifying*, and people will struggle with the last of their strength to clear the obstruction.

When used properly, the plastic Exit Bag causes a peaceful death; one that comes from (freely) breathing an atmosphere where there is no oxygen (*hypoxia*). With an Exit Bag, a person breathes easily and peacefully; the bag expands and contracts with each breath but there is very little oxygen present in the gas.

This is in stark contrast to the terror of suffocation and is why it is important *not to confuse* the peaceful hypoxic death that is possible when an Exit bag is used properly, with the grim death that results from an obstruction to the airways.

And this is why we should be wary of media reports that reinforce this confusion. For example, when referring in 2001 to the importation of Canadian Exit bags, the Murdoch press (*The Australian* newspaper) reported these bags as 'reminiscent of the Khmer Rouge's shopping bag executions in Cambodia's killing fields.' Such reports show a lack of understanding of the process and have damaged the image of the Exit Bag.

The Hypoxic Death

Hypoxia is the term meaning 'low oxygen', and a death that results from inhaling insufficient oxygen is a hypoxic death. While there are several ways this might occur, the common method used by those seeking a peaceful death is to suddenly immerse oneself in a non-oxygen environment. The simplest way to achieve this is by filling a plastic bag with an inert gas and then to quickly place this bag over one's head. To understand why the plastic Exit bag provides an easy and reliable way to die, a basic understanding of human physiology is helpful.

In normal everyday life, we live in an atmosphere that is 21% oxygen. Interestingly, when there is a decline in the level of oxygen in the air we are breathing, we do not experience any particular alarm or concern. As long as one can breathe easily, the sensation one experiences as the oxygen level drops is one of disorientation, confusion, lack of coordination and eventual loss of consciousness.

This experience is sometimes likened to being drunk (alcohol intoxication). If the oxygen level is too low death will result. Accidental hypoxic deaths are not uncommon and there are a number of scenarios that can bring them about.

One example is the sudden drop in oxygen level that occurs when an aeroplane depressurises at high altitude. This can lead to a rapid loss of consciousness and the death of all those in the plane.

When the plane de-pressurizes, one can still breath easily but there will be little oxygen in the inhaled air. This will cause a sudden drop in the dissolved oxygen in the blood reaching the brain, leading to loss of consciousness and death.

It is not uncommon for planes that have suddenly de-pressurized to travel on autopilot until they run out of fuel while everyone aboard has died. Witnesses (from planes sent to investigate) say that it often appears as though everyone on board has just gone to sleep.

Pneumonia is a more common cause of a hypoxic death. Its peaceful reputation led to its common description as the 'old person's friend'. While the air inhaled may contain the full 21% of oxygen, the inflammation of the lungs (caused by the pneumonic infection) makes it impossible for the necessary oxygen to be extracted. The blood reaching the brain will have less oxygen than that required for life, and a peaceful death often results.

The presence of an inert gas like Nitrogen or Helium in the Exit Bag dramatically speeds the process. When one exhales fully and then pulls down the Exit bag pre-filled with Nitrogen and takes a deep breath in one's lungs are filled with a gas in which there is very little oxygen. Blood passing the lungs on the way to the brain finds no oxygen available and when this blood with a low oxygen level reaches the brain, consciousness is rapidly lost, within one or two breaths. It is this lack of oxygen in the inhaled gas that causes death.

It is important to note that the inert gas does not interact with the body. Nitrogen, argon or helium have no taste or smell and quickly dissipate after death. While helium can be detected at autopsy, there is no test that can reveal the use of a nitrogen-filled Exit bag, making it particularly useful for folk who don't wish their cause of death to ever be established. (Of course this presupposes that the equipment will be removed before the body is 'discovered'.

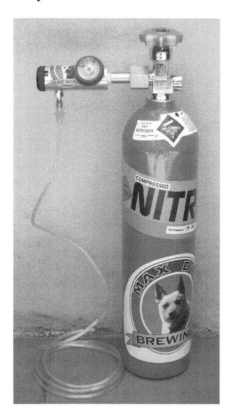

Fig 5.1: 380 litre 'Max Dog'
Nitrogen cylinder

The Role of Carbon Dioxide (CO_2)

In normal respiration, the human body uses oxygen and produces as waste the gas, carbon dioxide. Carbon dioxide is then removed from the body as we exhale. While the human body is relatively insensitive to falling levels of oxygen, it is *very* sensitive to any rise in the level of carbon dioxide in inhaled air.

When the body detects a slight increase of carbon dioxide in the air that we breathe, a warning message from the brain alerts the person. They will be roused and may react by gasping. If the person is using a plastic Exit bag, any rise in the level of carbon dioxide within the bag may result in the person struggling to pull the bag from their head. This reaction is known as a Hypercapnic (high carbon dioxide) Alarm Response.

Sleep Apnea provides an example of hypercapnic alarm. Here the person with sleep apnea snores so heavily that they deny themselves the oxygen they need. However, it is not the lowering of the oxygen level that alarms and wakes the person, but the accompanying rise in the level of carbon dioxide.

If the fall in oxygen were not accompanied by this rise in carbon dioxide, the Sleep Apneic would be far more likely to die. In the depressurized aircraft, the oxygen level drops but there is no accompanying rise in carbon dioxide, hence a peaceful death is the common outcome.

Aesthetic and Other Concerns

The image of a bag tied tightly around one's neck causing a grim death by obstructing the airway has turned many away from the plastic Exit Bag. Even at Exit International workshops, it is common for participants to voice their disgust at the Exit Bag, saying 'I don't like the thought of being found like that.'

Lisette Nigot rejected this method (see *Mademoiselle and the Doctor*, Chapter 1). Lisette likened the plastic Exit Bag to being 'wrapped like a piece of ham.' For Lisette and others, the main concern was one of aesthetics. Despite such concerns, if used correctly, the Exit Bag provides a simple, reliable and peaceful way of ending one's life.

A Peaceful Death

The best method of using an Exit Bag involves the use of an inert gas, such as Nitrogen, Helium or Argon.

The use of an inert gas is advocated because of its ability to create a space devoid of oxygen. This makes a peaceful death from hypoxia - lack of oxygen - possible in a relatively short space of time. The person only has the Exit Bag over their head for a matter of seconds until unconsciousness occurs, and there is almost no risk of a person experiencing an adverse reaction to a rising level of carbon dioxide within the Bag.

And this is why the Exit Bag, when combined with the steady flow of an inert gas like Nitrogen, is so effective. The flow of gas into the Exit Bag, displaces any residual or exhaled oxygen and flushes away any exhaled carbon dioxide. One does not need to wait for the oxygen inside the bag to be used up by the person wanting to die, it starts at 0% , and the gas flow ensures there is no associated build up of carbon dioxide.

There is *nothing* particularly special about the inert gas. Indeed, any gas that does not react with the body, is odourless and available in a compressed form would be suitable.

Most compressed gases are only available in high pressure cylinders which are rented from gas supply companies (like BOC Gases). These cylinders are available for lease ONLY, either short term or for an annual fee. The drawback with accessing a compressed gas this way is the paper trail that is generates. There is no anonymity. Commercial compressed gas cylinders are often large, heavy and difficult to transport. Suspicion might arise if an elderly or very sick person is seen leasing a cylinder from their local BOC gas outlet. If someone else were to collect the cylinder for them, this other person may well become legally implicated in assisting in a suicide. These concerns turned many people away from using high pressure, compressed inert gas with an Exit bag.

An exception is the introduction by Exit in 2012 of light-weight 'Max Dog' high pressure Nitrogen cylinders that one can purchase full with a suitable flow regulator. These aluminium cylinders weigh ~3Kg, contain ~400 litres of gas and can be purchased outright (with no paper trail) and then stored indefinitely for possible future use.

Low pressure disposable cylinders of Helium and Argon are also available and can be used effectively with the Exit Bag. As a result, the Exit Bag has undergone a significant rise in use as an end-of-life choice. In Australia, the US and UK, Helium is marketed in disposable "Balloon Time" containers so that balloons can be filled at home for parties (Fig 5.5 shows the two available sizes, 250 litre, and 420 litre), Argon is also available in disposable form, for use in welding applications (see fig 5.6).

The Optimal Gas Flow Rate

To achieve a peaceful hypoxic death with an inert gas and an Exit Bag, the optimal gas flow is one that flushes away exhaled carbon dioxide so this gas does not accumulate within the bag. This optimal gas flow also prevents the bag from heating up, but is slow enough so that useful flow will continue for > 20 minutes.

To determine the optimal flow Exit carried out experiments where different flow rates of air were admitted to a bag over a subject's head. The level of carbon dioxide within the bag was monitored using an RKI sampling gas detector.

Results for an 80 Kg male taken over a 5 minute period for two gas flow rates (5 & 15 l/min) are shown in Fig 5.2

For 15 l/min gas flow the level of carbon dioxide in the bag does not rise appreciably over the 5 minute period. With the low flow rate carbon dioxide level approached 5%, enough to make the subject uncomfortable and alarmed. A flow rate of ~15 l/min was seen as optimal.

When using Max Dog Nitrogen cylinders, the flow regulator can be set to 15 litres/ min and the gas will flow at this rate till the cylinder is exhausted (~400/15 or ~25 minutes, more than enough for a reliable and peaceful death)

When using disposable Balloon Time cylinders as a source of helium it can be difficult to control the flow of gas. The nylon tap provided with the cylinder is designed to fill party balloons. The tap is not designed to allow a more subtle gas flow rate. For use with an Exit bag, Exit recommends that the nylon fitting be discarded and replaced with Exit's brass jet flow fitting.

Using the Exit flow control kit on a standard 420 litre helium cylinder gives a useful operating time of ~20 minutes. This same fitting can be modified to control the flow of nitrogen from the filled LPG cylinder (Fig 5.6).

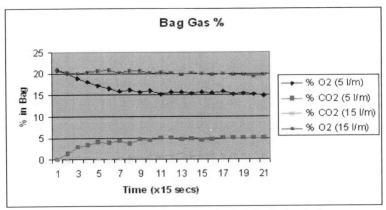

Fig 5.2: Exit Bag CO_2 & O_2 concentration lvels for the first 5 minutes

The Gas Source (Nitrogen, Helium or Argon)

1. Nitrogen and the Max Dog Delivery System

Nitrogen is a very common gas, making up ~ 80% of the air we breath. The gas is cheap, in no danger of running out, and readily available. It is not restricted and no questions are asked about why one would want a source of this gas, although one might say, if asked, that you are working on a nitrogen gas system for your home beer brew and want to achieve the fine bubbles and creamy head associated with Guinness stout (Nitrogen is used to aerate Guinness stout)

Since 2012, disposable cylinders filled with nitrogen are available from Max Dog Brewing. These high pressure cylinders containing ~400 litres of nitrogen.

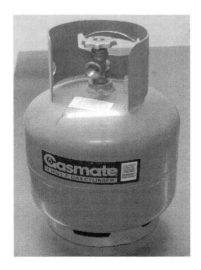
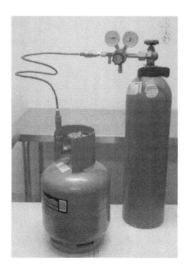

Fig 5.3: Filling a 4Kg LPG cylinder with 400 psi of Nitrogen

Prior to 2012, Exit suggested the use of LPG (liquid petroleum gas) cylinders as a possible container to store compressed nitrogen. These cylinders, which are designed to hold 4Kg of LPG, are easily obtained new and can be filled with nitrogen to a pressure of 3.3 MPa (or 480 psi). At ~400 psi there is ~ 250 litres of nitrogen in the tank and useful flow rates can be maintained for 15 to 20 minutes (Fig 5.6).

Problems associated with the safe filling of these tanks, and the need for some suitable regulation of pressure and flow control led to the abandonment of the LPG system and its replacement with the high pressure Max Dog Nitrogen system

Regulating the Flow of Nitrogen

Regulating the flow of nitrogen from the high pressure Max Dog cylinder is best achieved using a dedicated flow regulator (see Fig 5.4b). These regulators have a pressure gauge fitted that indicates the pressure in the cylinder, and a click setting to adjust the flow rate. The optimum flow rate fro a peaceful death (15 litres/ min) is one of the settings. The delivery hose to take the nitrogen to the Exit Bag fits directly onto the regulator outlet.

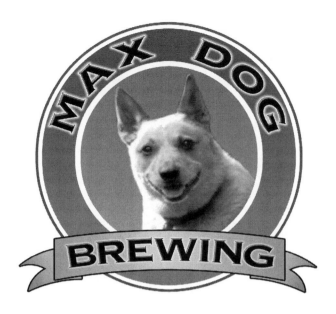

The Max Dog Nitrogen System

Max Dog is an international retailer of Nitrogen based in Adelaide, South Australia.

The Max Dog nitrogen system consists of 2.8 litre alloy cylinders filled to a pressure of 13.1 MPa (1800 psi) (See Fig 5.61a). The cylinders weigh ~3 Kg and full they contain 390 litres of nitrogen. When the gas is delivered at the optimum 15 litres/min, a full cylinder provides 26 minutes of constant gas flow into the Exit bag. This is more than enough for a peaceful death. For details see Fig 5.10a, or visit: *http://www.maxdogbrewing.com*

One useful aspect of the Nitrogen System is the fact that the cylinders can be topped up if there is leakage of nitrogen over time (the disposable Helium and Argon cylinders cannot be refilled). Note: The pressure measurement needed to establish that a cylinder is full is provided by the gauge on the regulator provided.

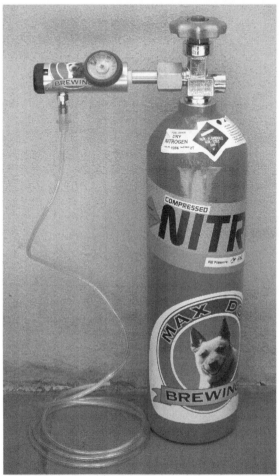

Fig 5.4
(a) 400 litre Max Dog cylinder ready to connect to Exit Bag
(b) Max Dog Nitrogen flow regulatorshowing the guage to indicate if the cylinder is fullof Nitrogen and the çlick'flow setting (shown set to 15 litres/min)

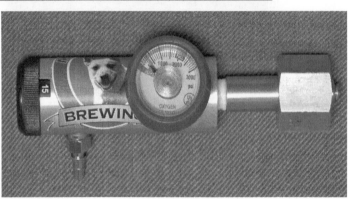

2. Helium

Disposable, compressed Helium comes as part of a Balloon Kit manufactured in the US. These kits are designed to provide an instant system to fill helium party balloons and contain a light-weight cylinder of helium, a packet of party balloons (30 or 50 depending upon the size cylinder) and tie ribbon. The Kits can be purchased outright, with cash, leaving no paper trail.

In Nth America, Balloon Time canisters are available at Amazon's online store (*http://www.latimes.com/news/nationworld/ world/la-fg-mexico-rehab-attack4-2009sep04,0,5425770.story*).

In the UK, Balloon Time canisters are available at Toys R Us at: *http://www.toysrus.co.uk/Toys-R-Us/Outdoor-and-Sports/Trampolines-and-Inflatables/Balloon-Time-Helium-Cylinder%280101864%29?searchP osition=8* and at Tescos at: *https://www.tescoparty.com/ShowProducts. aspx?PageID=453*

In Australia and New Zealand many, but not all, Spotlight stores stock Balloon Time canisters.

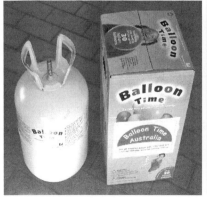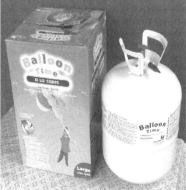

Fig 5.5: Packages disposable Helium containers: Left - 420 litre, Right - 250 Litre

There are two sizes of cylinder available, a larger cylinder which contains 420 litres (14.9 cubic feet) of compressed helium at a pressure of ~ 1.5MPa or a smaller cylinder that contains 250 litres (8.8 cubic feet) of compressed helium at a similar pressure. (Fig 5.5).

While there is enough helium in a small cylinder for a peaceful death, close control of the gas flow rate in the small cylinders is essential.

The larger 420 litre cylinders give greater margin for error and are preferred for this reason. This cylinder will produce a usable stream of gas that will run for approximately 20 minutes; more than enough time for a peaceful death to occur. Useful flow rates are obtained from either cylinder (>5 litres/min for 15 minutes with the small cylinder, and 25 minutes with the larger - see Fig 5.5a).

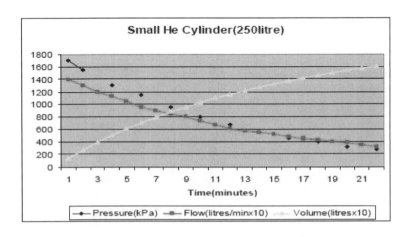

Fig 5.5a: Flow Rate, Pressure and Volume of Helium with Time for 420 & 250 litre Cylinders using the Exit Gas Control Jet Assembly

3. Argon

Small non-refillable bottles of compressed Argon for use in welding applications are available (see fig 5.6). The cylinders are small (~ 1 litre) and light (~ 1Kg) and the argon is stored at relatively high pressure (~ 6000 kPa or 900 psi). A regulator designed for use with the cylinders is available and allows good flow control.

It is important to note though that with a flat rate of gas flow of around 8 litres/ min there is only a useful period of 8 to 10 minutes.

Once the argon gas fills the Exit bag there is little time for reflection!

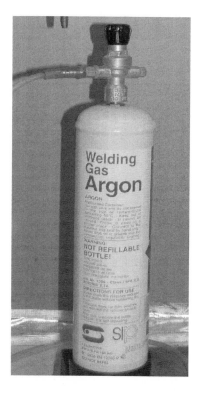

Fig 5.6: 60 litre disposable Argon cylinder

The Exit Bag

The Exit plastic bag is the bag which is filled with the inert gas. The bag is designed to enable simple filling with no contamination with oxygen, providing a straight forward way for one to suddenly immerse oneself in inert gas.

1. Making an Exit Bag

While different people make slightly different bags, the standard Exit Bag involves a plastic bag of:

- a reasonable size
- a suitable soft plastic
- a neck band of elastic that allows the bag to make a snug, but not tight, fit around a person's neck

In the past, Exit Bags have been able to be purchased from organizations such as Right to Die Canada. As the original inventors of the Bag, Right to Die Canada were active for many years in their manufacture and sale and for a while provided a mail order service for their members.

For a short period in 2001 and again in 2011, Exit International also sold Exit bags. However, with the experience of Sharlotte Hydorn of the Gladd organisation in California in early 2011 (her home was raided by the police and FBI who seized all manner of property) fresh in our minds Exit has revised its position for the time being at least. See: *http://bit.ly/qunUq0*

In recent years, it has been Nurse Betty who has taught readers of this book how to stay safe in the law and make their own Exit bags.

To make an Exit Bag, several items are needed (see Fig 5.7)

- Plastic bag - polyester 'oven bag' available in supermarkets is a good size (Large 35cm x 48cm) 'A & B'
- 1 metre of 10 mm wide elastic, 'D'
- 1 toggle to adjust elastic length
- 1 roll of 20mm sticky tape 'C' (Micropore or equivalent)
- 1 small roll of ~ 35 mm plastic duct tape
- Pair of sharp scissors

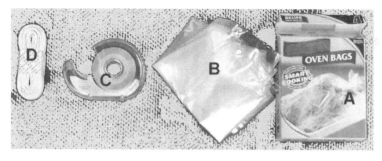

Fig 5.7 Items used to construct an Exit Bag

Construction   (See Fig 5.8 & *Do it with Betty* video)

1. Lay the bag out on a flat surface and folded back ~ 25mm (1") around the open end (A-B)
2. Make a 25mm cut in the folded polyester
3. Lay the elastic (C) inside the fold and had the two ends exit through this cut
4. Tape completely along the folded edge of the plastic with the sticky tape
5. Place a cut in a ~ 60mm piece of duct tape and fold this over the exiting elastic to strengthen this part of the bag
6. Thread a small wire tie through two cuts in another piece (~50mm) of duct tape and stick this to the inside of the bag ~ 15cm up from the elastic (E). This can be used to secure the plastic helium hose inside the bag.
7. The toggle (D) is then threaded onto the two ends of the elastic to complete the bag (Fig 5.9)

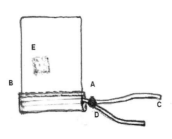

Fig 5.8: Exit Bag Manufacture

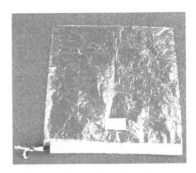

Fig 5.9: The completed Exit Bag

Gas Flow Control

No matter which gas is used a flow velocity of ~ 15 l/min is needed to prevent the accumulation of CO_2 in the Exit bag. Exit has investigated several methods of controlling gas flow.

• For high pressure cylinders of nitrogen (Max Dog or equivalent) or helium, regulation is essential. Flow regulators are provided with the Max Dog system or can be purchased from gas providers. The Max Dog regulator shown in Fig 5.9.2 gives the pressure of nitrogen in the cylinder, and allows the output flow rate to be set at 15 litres/min. Using this regulator, flow rate is constant throughout the hypoxic death.

• For disposable 'Balloon Time' helium cylinders at pressures of 1.7MPa, Exit has designed gas flow control fittings expressly for this purpose (Fig 5.11). These fittings give an initial flow rate of ~20 litres/min when the tap is opened fully. Exit helium flow fittings are available

• at: *http://www.exitinternationalstore.com/Flow-Control-Fitting-Gauge-HF.htm*

For the low-pressure nitrogen system described (Fig 5.3) with filling pressures of 2.8MPa (400psi), a standard LPG regulator restricting the outlet pressure to ~ 2.8kPa with a jet (size ~2mm) will provide the appropriate flow rate.

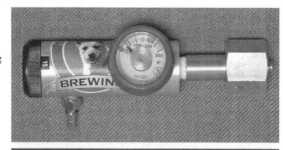

Fig 5.9.2
High pressure Max Dog
nitrogen regulator with
click flow rate output

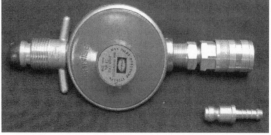

Fig 5.9.1
LPG regulator
and 2mm jet
used to control
nitrogen flow

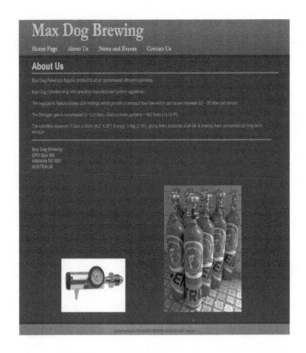

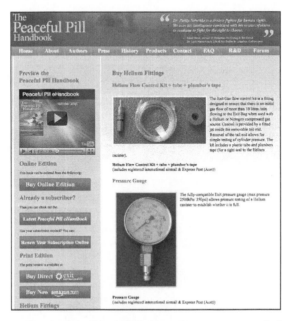

Fig 5.10a Max Dog nitrogen cylinder and regulator order page www.maxdogbrewing.com.au:
Fig 5.10b Helium flow fittings purchase page www.peacefulpill.com

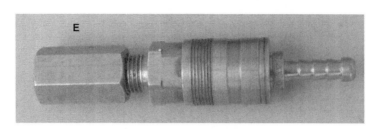

Fig 5.11: The Exit Helium flow control fitting

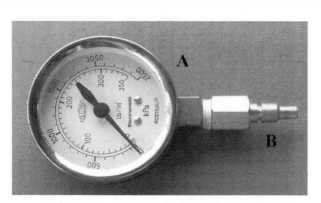

Fig 5.12: Pressure gauge used to check if gas cylinder is full

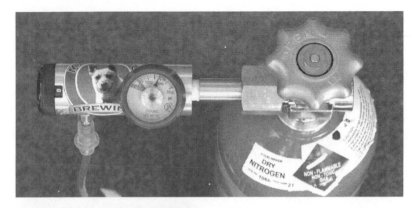

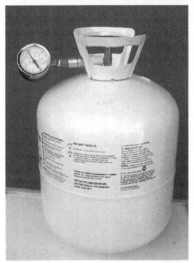

Fig 5.13:
(a) Checking the pressure of a full max Dog nitrogen cylinder. Flow 0 l/min, Pressure 13MPa

(b)Helium cylinder with pressure gauge attached to flow control assembly. Full pressure 250psi or 1.7MPa

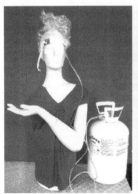
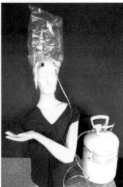
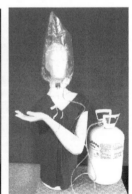

Fig 5.14: Positioning, inflating & Using the Exit Bag with Helium

Testing the Pressure of the Gas in the Cylinder

With the Exit bag method, it is important to establish that there is sufficient gas available for a peaceful hypoxic death. For compressed gas in cylinders, the easiest way of ensuring this is to measure the pressure. This is particularly important for cylinders that have been kept in storage for long periods.

When using the Max Dog high pressure nitrogen system, the pressure will be shown by the gauge on the regulator. To measure this, switch the regulator flow rate to 0 litres/min and open the cylinder to read the pressure. This should be ~12MPa (1750psi) (see Fig 5.13a)

For Balloon Time helium cylinders a pressure gauge that fits the flow control makes testing the pressure simple. A full cylinder should have a pressure of ~ 1.7MPa (250 psi). Some of these cylinders have been found to have faulty taps and to be near empty on purchase. A suitable pressure gauge is available from *http://bit.ly/9swOxk* (see Fig 5.13b, 5.10b & 5.12).

For a LPG cylinder, the pressure should be ~2800kPa (400psi). If a regulator and large jet are to be used with the LPG cylinder, pressure measurements must be made upstream of the regulator.

Gas Purity

Exit occasionally receives reports of failures by people using Exit Bags with helium. Although this information is sketchy, the reports are of people breathing the gas inside the bag for some minutes with no loss of consciousness. This has not been reported with nitrogen. Contamination of Balloon Time helium has been suggested as an explanation.

The only possible contamination that could produce this effect would be the addition of a significant quantity of oxygen to the helium. The introduction of 10% of oxygen would have no effect on the marketed use of the gas - balloons filled with this mixture would float - but this gas would fail in an Exit bag.

Every year, Exit tests new Balloon Time helium cylinders. The results of these tests have been reassuring with no evidence of significant contamination.

Typical Helium gas analysis:
O_2 ~0.4%, CO_2 <0.01%,
CO <0.1ppm,   Hydrocarbons ~ 40ppm.

Note: The gas used in these failed attempts has not been tested.

Note: Exit has been in contact with the manufacturers of *Balloon Time* helium cylinders. We have been assured that if oxygen were to be added to their helium cylinders it would be noted prominently on the cylinder.

Connecting the Cylinder to the Exit Bag

To use the Exit Bag with an inert gas, one needs to connect the gas cylinder to the Exit bag. Plastic tubing (standard 2 metre oxygen tubing with soft connectors) is suitable for this purpose and comes included with the Max Dog nitrogen system, and the Exit helium flow fitting. The tubing is tightly fitted to the Max Dog regulator outlet, or the tail-end on the helium flow control fitting. The other end is then stuck to the inside of the Exit bag with Micropore tape. It is recommended to test that the attachment of the tube to the flow fitting and to the Exit bag is secure and not easily dislodged.

The Procedure

The goal for this method is to produce a reliable, quick and peaceful death from hypoxia. There are 3 stages in this process and these are shown in the Video (Betty and the Exit Bag) and in fig 5.14.

• Adjust the elastic in neck of the bag so that it is a firm fit around the human neck. Then place the bag on the head across the forehead. Crush the bag down onto the head to exclude all air then open the tap on the Helium bottle. The flow of Helium at ~15 l/min fills the bag in about a minute.

• When the bag is filled with gas the Helium will begin to leak around the elastic while the bag remains fully inflated. A quick look in the mirror will enable the bag to be correctly positioned and full of Helium.

• To bring about a peaceful death, a person would exhale totally (fully empty their lungs) and hold their breath while pulling the bag down over their head. When the bag is over the head and snugly around the neck, they would take the deepest breath possible. Loss of consciousness will occur almost immediately - within one or two breaths. Death occurs few minutes later.

Who should not use the Exit Bag

For a peaceful death one must be able to fully exhale and inhale. This allows the rapid exchange of the air in the lungs with the gas in the bag. Some respiratory diseases can make this difficult or impossible.

For example, people with emphysema or chronic obstructive airways disease should be aware of possible problems if they attempt to use this method. If the gas exchange cannot take place quickly, the time before consciousness is lost can be unacceptably long and result in panic. This phenomena may explain some of the reports of unexplained failures using this method described in the "Gas Purity" section.

Cleaning Away - The Affect of Inert Gas on the Body

The use of an inert gas with an Exit Bag produces *no* changes in the body that can be seen or found on initial inspection. In 2007 forensic laboratory tests were developed to establish the presence of gases like Helium, Argon and Neon in the lungs of the deceased.

In 2009, the first report of the use of this technique in establishing the cause of death of an Exit member was noted. Such testing is uncommon and it remains true that if there is no evidence of an Exit bag or gas cylinder having being used, it is likely that the death will be certified as natural. The exception is Nitrogen.

If Nitrogen is used for a hypoxic death, and if the Exit bag and tube is removed, no conclusions can be drawn from detecting its presence. The Exit Bag with nitrogen is the only method of a peaceful and dignified death which provides total undetectability.

Concluding Comments

The Exit Bag with Inert Gas is an end of life method that is reliable, simple and does not involve illegal drugs or equipment. Nevertheless, the method demands substantial preparation. A disposable gas cylinder needs to be purchased, along with the requisite connections, tubing and a Bag must be made.

Technique is also important and a certain degree of physical dexterity is required. On the downside, the need for so much equipment and the unaesthetic nature of placing a bag over one's head prevents many people from even considering this method.

THE RP TEST SCORE – Exit Bag + Inert gas

Reliability   (R = 8/10)
The method is reliable but technique is important
and a degree of coordination and dexterity is required

Peacefulness   (P = 7/10)
Considered "peaceful" partly because the loss
of consciousness comes quickly. There is the
sensation of "air hunger" and alarm

Availability   (A = 5/5)
All components are readily available

Preparation   (Pr = 1/5)
Considerable assembly and "setting up" of equipment

Undetectability   (U = 5/5)
If all equipment is removed detection is rare. If Nitrogen is the gas used the method is totally undetectable.

Speed   (Sp = 5/5)
Loss of consciousness comes quickly

Safety   (Sa = 5/5)
The method presents no danger to others

Storage   (St = 5/5)
Components do not deteriorate with time. Pressure testing can readily establish that the cylinder is full

Total RP Score   **41/50 (82%)**

THE RP TEST SCORE – Exit Bag + Inert gas

Criteria	Score
Reliability	*8/10*
Peacefulness	*7/10*
Availability	*5/5*
Preparation	*1/5*
Undetectability	*5/5*
Speed	*5/5*
Safety	*5/5*
Storage	*5/5*
Total	*41 (82%)*

Chapter 5: Frequently Asked Questions

• *Can a face-mask be used instead of the Exit Bag?*

Common, inexpensive facemasks are often used to deliver oxygen to patients. They are usually held in place by elastic which covers the nose and mouth with oxygen delivered through a plastic tube attached to the base of the mask. There is no attempt to seal the mask and face. The purpose is simply to increase the concentration of oxygen breathed above the usual 21%.

In contrast, the Exit Bag produces rapid loss of consciousness by ensuring that NO oxygen is inhaled. To achieve this using a mask, flow delivery flow rates of at least 20 litres/sec would be required to reduce the chance of oxygen contamination during inspiration (ie. 100 times that necessary with the Exit Bag!).

While technically possible, a large diameter delivery hose would be needed along with a gas source very much greater than the 420 litre Balloon Time cylinders. Risky and not recommended.

• *Do I need to connect 2 Balloon Time Helium Cylinders to ensure Sufficient Gas is Available?*

No, this is not necessary if the flow of gas is regulated using the Exit flow control fitting. With the gas flow regulated, even the smaller (250 litre) Balloon Time cylinder will provide sufficient gas flow, ensuring there is no build up of carbon dioxide in the bag for at least 15 minutes (Fig 5.4). This is more than enough time for a peaceful death.

If the tube is to be connected directly to the cylinder with no gas flow regulation (other than the cylinder on/off tap), multiple cylinders should be employed.

6

Carbon Monoxide

Introduction

Carbon Monoxide (CO) is one of the most lethal gases known. Its toxicity is due to its ability to strongly bind with haemoglobin which greatly reduces the oxygen-carrying capacity of a person's blood. Areas of the brain sensitive to ischaemia (low oxygen level) are affected severely and a rapid, peaceful death is the common result. The gas is particularly dangerous, as it is a colourless, odourless and a non-irritating gas. Without specialized monitoring equipment, there is no way of knowing that carbon monoxide is present.

Death by poisoning from carbon monoxide can be reliable, quick and peaceful, provided the concentration of the inhaled gas is sufficiently high. In the 1990s, Dr Jack Kevorkian helped more than 100 seriously ill people to end their lives peacefully, nearly half of whom used carbon monoxide. Dr Kevorkian used a cylinder of compressed carbon monoxide (9% CO in Nitrogen). The person wanting to die switched on the gas at the cylinder and breathed through a loose-fitting face mask. A few deep breaths of the carbon monoxide-nitrogen mixture and the person lost consciousness and died quickly. Dr Kevorkian would then switch off the gas and remove the cylinder and face mask. Those present at these deaths described the effectiveness and peacefulness of the approach.

PPM [CO]	Time	Symptoms
35	8 hours	Maximum exposure allowed by OSHA in the workplace over an eight hour period.
200	2-3 hours	Mild headache, fatigue, nausea and dizziness.
400	1-2 hours	Serious headache-other symptoms intensify. Life threatening after 3 hours.
800	45 minutes	Dizziness, nausea and convulsions. Unconscious within 2 hours. Death within 2-3 hours.
1600	20 minutes	Headache, dizziness and nausea. Death within 1 hour.
3200	5-10 minutes	Headache, dizziness and nausea. Death within 1 hour.
6400	1-2 minutes	Headache, dizziness and nausea. Death within 25-30 minutes.
12,800	1-3 minutes	Rapid Death

Table 6.1 Effect of carbon monoxide exposure

It is important to establish that monoxide concentration is high enough as periods of time spent in sub-lethal gas levels can lead to serious irreparable damage. From the accompanying table (Table 6.1) it is clear that although death will occur at much lower levels, if one is in the environment for some time, it is strongly recommended that concentrations greater than 1% (10,000 ppm) are generated by the method chosen.

There are often no specific clinical findings to identify this agent as the cause of death, although occasionally the red colouration of 'venous' blood gives a flushed pink colour to the skin of the corpse. This colouration may indicate the cause of death to an examining doctor and its presence will be detected at autopsy. If it is important that the death look 'natural' (and 'suicide' not be stated on the death certificate), then poisoning by carbon monoxide may not be the best choice.

Testing the Concentration of Carbon Monoxide

To ensure that the monoxide concentration is sufficiently high for a peaceful death, it is wise to test the gas concentration. To do this one needs an appropriate meter capable of reading carbon monoxide concentration levels.

Exit has tested several meters for this purpose. The cheapest monitors have only a warning light set to alarm when levels of 50ppm are exceeded. These are of limited use.

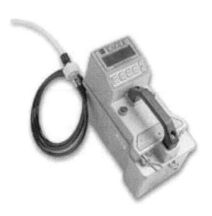
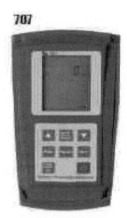
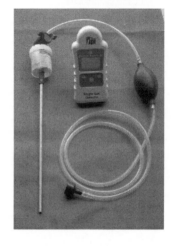

Fig 6.2
a) RKI sampling multi-gas meter
b) TPI 707 high level monoxide analyser
c) TPI 770 monitor with sampling probe

Gauges with a digital readout of up to to 1000 ppm (0.1%) can be easily obtained. It is advisable to have a sampling facility on the gauge so that the level produced can be sampled before using this method. Sampling gauges can be modified with a 10:1 reduction, so that levels up to and greater than 1% can be measured.

Gauges used by Exit are shown in Fig 6.2. The multi-gas sampling meter (RKI Eagle) enables the monitoring of carbon monoxide levels, carbon dioxide levels as well as the concentration of available oxygen. This gauge retails for over US$2000 and is primarily used as a research tool. A smaller hand-held device (TPI model 701 carbon monoxide analyser) that measures aspirated gas of up to 10,000 ppm is also shown. This useful gauge costs ~ US$600. A cheaper TPI gauge used by Exit with a modified 10:1 sampling probe (TPI model 770) costs ~US$200.

Sources of Carbon Monoxide

From Commercial Gas Suppliers:
Cylinders of compressed carbon monoxide, either as the pure gas or as a mixture (eg 5% in Nitrogen) are available from scientific gas supply companies. There are no special restrictions but an account will be needed. Table 6.1 lists some available packaging for pure compressed carbon monoxide from BOC.
http://www.boc.com/

Cylinders of special gas mixtures that contain lethal levels of monoxide are also used as source gases for some industrial lasers (eg 6% CO in gas used in the Rofin CO_2 slab laser).
http://www.linde-electronics.eu/sg/mixsg/lasermix__690_en.html

Carbon Monoxide (CO)

a toxic, flammable, colourless and odourless gas

Grade	Minimum Purity (%)	Cylinder Size	Contents	Pressure (kPa)*	BAR	Valve	Equipment Recommended
Australia							
Chemically Pure Grade 2.5 Gas Code 156	99.5	LB (A)	0.05 m³	10300	103	CGA170	Regulators for CGA170 See Section on Regulators
		1A (G)	4.8 m³	11300	113	CGA350	Regulators for CGA350 See Section on Regulators
		D	0.66 m³	7000	70	Type 20	Regulators for Type 20 See Section on Regulators
		2 (E)	1.8 m³	1100	11	CGA350	Regulators for CGA350 See Section on Regulators
		200	4.85 m³	11300	113		
		300	7.36 m³	11300	113		

Table 6.3. Compressed CO cylinder sizes

Vehicle Exhaust Gas:

Carbon Monoxide is produced as an exhaust gas from internal combustion engines. The concentration of the monoxide in the exhaust gas varies, depending on a number of factors and establishing this is critical.

Using Formic Acid:

Carbon Monoxide is produced by a chemical reaction that occurs when the formic acid (HCOOH) is broken down into water (H_2O) and carbon monoxide (CO). The catalyst for this breakdown is concentrated sulphuric acid. The sulphuric acid remains chemically unchanged but is diluted by the water released.

Monoxide generation ceases when all of the formic acid is broken down, or when the sulphuric acid becomes too dilute to catalyze the reaction. Heat is generated in the reaction and this can lead to traces of formic and sulphuric acid in the emerging carbon monoxide. One mole of formic acid (46gm) will produce ~22 litres of carbon monoxide.

The chemical equation is: $HCOOH \Rightarrow H_2O + CO$

Using Oxalic Acid:

Concentrate sulphuric acid can be used to breakdown anhydrous oxalic acid to produce carbon monoxide (and carbon dioxide). Again the sulphuric acid remains chemically unchanged but is diluted by the water produced in the reaction. Less heat is generated in the reaction and there is less likelihood of contamination with vapour from the sulphuric acid. One mole of oxalic acid (~90gm) produces equal molar amounts of carbon dioxide and carbon dioxide.

The chemical equation is: $HO_2CCO_2H \Rightarrow H_20 + CO_2 + CO$

Using Carbon (charcoal):
The incomplete oxidation of carbon can produce copious amounts of carbon monoxide. As the oxygen available to a charcoal fire decreases the production of carbon dioxide decreases and carbon monoxide increases.

The chemical equation is: $2C + O2 \Rightarrow 2CO$

Using Zinc and Calcium Carbonate:
Powdered zinc can be mixed with calcium carbonate and heated to produce carbon monoxide, along with calcium and zinc oxide. Heat is needed for the process and this offers the opportunity of controlling the process (using an electrical heater).

The chemical equation is: $Zn + CaCO_3 \rightarrow ZnO + CaO + CO$

Using Vehicle Exhaust Gas as a Source of Carbon Monoxide

Internal combustion engines produce a small percentage of carbon monoxide in the exhaust gas. If this gas is inhaled, death will result. Piping the gas into the car, or running the car in a closed shed are common approaches. In all cases, though, the carbon monoxide will be mixed with a large amount of other foul-smelling exhaust products. One of the benefits of using this gas, peacefulness, is lost.

Older cars tend to produce the highest levels of exhaust carbon monoxide. With the introduction of unleaded petrol in the 80s, there have been controls on the monoxide levels in exhaust gases to meet environmental standards. Since 1997 new cars can emit no more that 10% of the levels of carbon monoxide acceptable in 1976. Mandatory catalytic convertors oxidize most of the produced carbon monoxide to form carbon dioxide.

Despite these significant changes in the emission levels of carbon monoxide, motor vehicle exhaust gas suicides continue to occur at a surprisingly high rate. Indeed, in the period from 1976 to 1995 the rate of exhaust gas suicides in some countries increased faster than the rate of motor vehicle registrations (Routley & Ozanne-Smith, 1998). Possible explanations include the fact that idling motors do not necessarily comply with international standards. Additionally, catalytic convertors do not function when cold. Rather, they require several minutes to warm from a cold start. Of significance though is the increasing number of failed suicide attempts from breathing exhaust gas reported in this period.

This is not to say that the motor car cannot be used as a source of carbon monoxide to effect a reliable death, but there are problems associated with the method. One concern is the mechanical connection of the exhaust to the hose carrying gas to the car. Many modern vehicles have elliptical exhaust outlets. Coupling the exhaust to a round hose, often using plastic tape, can cause problems because of the heat of exhaust gas. If the tape or tube melts or is destroyed by the heat, failure is likely. Fig 6.4 shows a carefully engineered system using metal connections and clamps and heat resistant tubing.

This approach demands meticulous attention to detail and testing

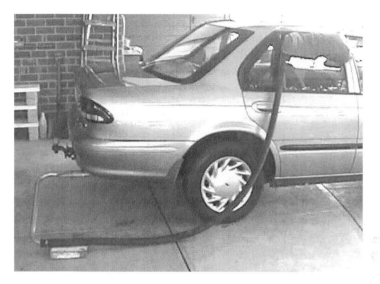

Fig 6.4. The car as a carbon monoxide source

is strongly recommended. A carbon monoxide meter should be used for testing. The meter should be placed on the front seat. The car should then be run using the planned setup. The meter can be watched safely from outside the car. The meter reading will soon show if the system will work. If the meter moves quickly off-scale (>500ppm), the method is unlikely to fail. If the meter struggles to rise, even when the motor is started cold and allowed to idle, the system should be avoided.

In addition, careful planning is required to avoid the possibility of intervention. A car running with a hose fed into the back window will almost certainly attract attention. And, even if effective, sitting in an environment of hot, foul smelling, burnt engine waste, just to make use of the tiny percentage of monoxide present, is an unpleasant way to die. In Exit's research of our elderly members' attitudes, only a small number showed interest in using exhaust carbon monoxide.

Making Carbon Monoxide (the COGen)

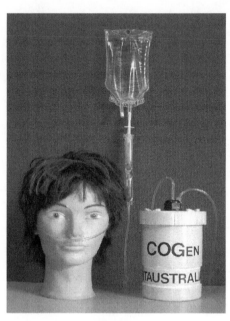

Fig 6.5
The early CoGen

For over a decade, Exit International has investigated the use of carbon monoxide. Since the compressed gas is difficult to source, Exit has developed generators that produce the carbon monoxide gas when and as required. The first carbon monoxide generator (the COGen) made use of the chemical reaction (catalytic breakdown) that takes place when formic acid is added to sulphuric acid.

In the original model (Fig 6.5) the formic acid was placed in an intravenous bag and allowed to drip into the reaction chamber containing the sulphuric acid. The gas produced was then fed to the mannequin using nasal prongs. Filmmaker Janine Hosking recorded this first demonstration at Exit's laboratory in late 2002, and the sequence was shown in the film *Mademoiselle and the Doctor*.

Since that time other methods of carbon monoxide generation have been investigated. Methods include the partial oxidation of carbon (charcoal), the reduction and catalytic conversion of oxalic acid, and the reaction between powdered zinc and calcium carbonate.

How the COGen Works

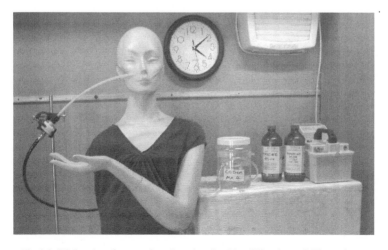

Fig 6.6. COGen 4 on fume cupboard test bench with acid bottles and CO monitor

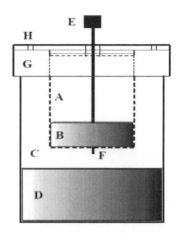

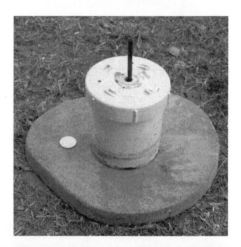

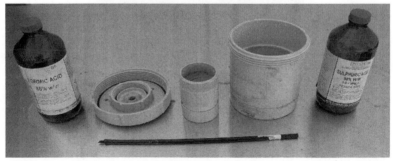

Fig 6.7 The COGen & acids

The COGen consists of two PVC chambers ('A' & 'C', Fig 6.7). The inner chamber "A' is mounted to the screw lid of the larger outer 10cm (3.9 inch) container and has a drip exit 'F' in its base. The drip rate is controlled by a screw 'E'.

150 ml of 85% formic acid is placed in chamber ('A') with the control-valve shut.

250ml of concentrated sulphuric acid (98%) is placed in the outer chamber 'D' and the COGen assembled.

Opening the screw 'E' allows the formic acid to drip into the concentrated sulphuric acid. Copious amounts of carbon monoxide are released and exit the chamber through vent holes in the lid 'H'.

The Video shows the COGen being armed and placed in a small car. The carbon monoxide concentration in the car was continuously sampled with a probe positioned near the head of the mannequin. The graph (Fig 6.8) shows the measured concentration in ppm, plotted over the first 30 minutes. Lethal concentrations were reached a few minutes after switching on the generator. A peak level of ~3% CO was recorded.

Sourcing the Acids

Concentrated sulphuric acid (98%) can be purchased from chemical suppliers or at hardware stores where it is sold as a drain cleaner. Concentrated laboratory sulphuric acid is an oily clear liquid, whereas the drain-cleaner sulphuric acid can be dark brown in colour because of additives, but this does not effect the generator's operation.

Formic acid is available from chemical supply companies.

Home hobbyists use formic acid in tanning or bee-keeping. Formic acid can also be purchased online through chemical supply websites.

Oxalic acid is used as rust and stain cleaner and can be purchased from hardware stores.

Safety Note

Concentrated formic and sulphuric acids are corrosive liquids. They should be kept secured in glass or polyethylene containers (plastic soft drink/ soda bottles are not suitable). When using sulphuric acid, rubber gloves should be worn along with eye-protecting goggles and a face-splash protector. Spills of acids on to the skin should be washed off immediately with copious amounts of water. If either of these acids gets in the eyes, wash the eyes continuously for several minutes and then seek medical assistance.

Generating Carbon Monoxide using a Charcoal Burner

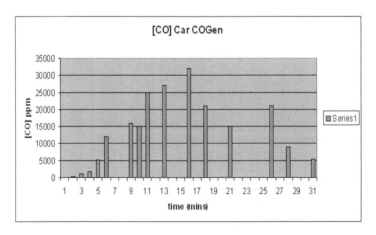

Table 6.8 CO concentration with time using COGen in a vehicle

This method of generation is commonly used as it is simple to set up and all necessary items are readily obtained. A charcoal burner can made from a steel container or by using a brazier or using a pre-packaged charcoal BBQ grill.

If you make your own burner, obtain good quality charcoal to reduce the level of unwanted smoke. You will also need a car, or other small room that can be sealed.

In the series of experiments carried out by Exit, a small pre-packaged charcoal burner was set alight and placed on the floor in a small car. The level of carbon monoxide inside the car was continuously monitored.

Other tests were carried out using a sealed 20ft shipping container as the closed environment. A brazier was loaded with 1.5 Kgm of good quality charcoal which was then set alight and placed in the centre of the floor. The container doors were shut (see Fig 6.10). Again, the carbon monoxide concentration within the container was continuously sampled from outside using a sampling probe.

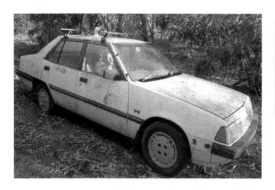
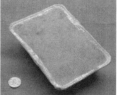

Fig 6.9 Test vehicle with BBQ charcoal burner

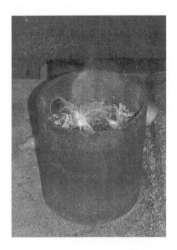 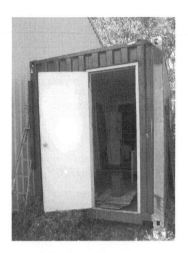

Fig 6.10. Charcoal burner.brazier and test shipping container

NOTE: It is stressed that carbon monoxide is an extremely lethal gas. A person wishing to end their life using this gas should not have others near them. This is one disadvantage of using carbon monoxide.

If carbon monoxide is used, place a warning sign in a prominent position to prevent any accidental exposure to other people.

Conclusion

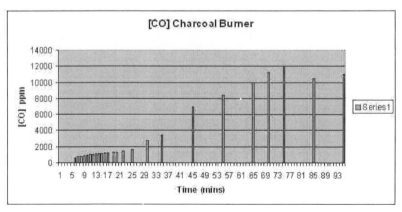

Table 6.11. CO concentration with time in test shipping container

Carbon Monoxide can provide a person with a peaceful death. The gas can be obtained in a variety of ways ranging from simple burners to more sophisticated generating devices. Tests should be made to ensure that concentrations of over 1% can be established.

Most interest in this method has come from those who reject the taking of drugs orally (eg. for fear of vomiting) and by others who reject the use of helium because of the need for a plastic bag to be placed over one's head. The COGen addresses these concerns.

Exit RP Test for Carbon Monoxide

The method loses points in the subcategories of Preparation, Undetectability and Safety. Preparation is not simple (Pr=1), there is equipment present at the death, and if using a COGen preparation with concentrated acids requires care. This method may be detectable on inspection of the body (U=2), and can present some risk to others (Sa=1).

Criteria	Score
Reliability	*8/10*
Peacefulness	*7/10*
Availability	*3/5*
Preparation	*1/5*
Undetectability	*1/5*
Speed	*5/5*
Safety	*1/5*
Storage	*4/5*
Total	*30 (60%)*

Cyanide

The death of Spaniard Ramon Sampedro in 1998 and the subsequent award-winning film *The Sea Inside* has focused attention on the use of cyanide as an effective means by which a seriously ill person can put an end to their suffering.

Sampedro, a quadriplegic since a diving accident at age 26, ended his life by drinking a glass of water in which soluble potassium cyanide had been dissolved. He died quickly, and peacefully. Many people who have seen *The Sea Inside* have asked why these cyanide salts are not more frequently used by those who are seriously ill to provide a peaceful death. In this chapter we explain some of the difficulties involved in using cyanide and provide some answers. It is not unreasonable to expect that the use of cyanide will increase in the future, and it may yet become an acceptable form of the 'Peaceful Pill'.

Some background to cyanide

In 1814, the carbon-nitrogen (CN) 'radical' common to a number of chemical substances was isolated and given the name 'cyanogen' by the French chemist Joseph Gay Lussac. The subsequent name 'the blue generator' referred to the place of the CN radical in a number of chemicals that were used as blue dyes; the Prussian Blue of blueprints (iron ferro cyanide) is perhaps the best known. In many of these compounds, the CN radical is so tightly bound that the substances are relatively non-toxic.

With the discovery of substances where the CN radical was not so tightly bound - the gas hydrogen cyanide, hydrocyanic acid, and simple salts like potassium and sodium cyanide - it was soon realised that cyanide was extremely toxic to animal cells. By destroying the mitochondria, an essential element within each cell, the CN radical caused rapid cellular death.

In 1921, cyanide gas (hydrogen cyanide, HCN) was proposed as a humane method of execution and led to the passage of the 'Humane Death Bill' in Nevada. The gas was first used to execute Gee Jon in 1924. Since that time nearly 1000 people have died in the execution gas chambers in the US. All chambers used the same method to produce cyanide gas. Pellets of sodium cyanide were dropped into sulphuric acid to release the gas which then enveloped the prisoner.

Hydrogen cyanide is a volatile liquid and can be stabilised and absorbed onto a substrate. In this form (Zyclon B), it was used by the Nazi's during the Holocaust. Originally developed as an insecticide, the pellets were kept in sealed containers and released as HCN gas when the pellets came into contact with air.

Today, cyanide compounds are widely used in industry. Vast quantities of the cyanide salts are produced for use in the gold mining, metallurgy, electroplating and photographic industries. Their toxicity is well known and despite the large quantities used, they remain heavily restricted and difficult to obtain.

Can Cyanide provide a peaceful and reliable death?

Those watching the cinematographic depiction of Sampedro's death would have cause to believe that a death resulting from the ingestion of cyanide salts is peaceful. Unfortunately, not all reports of cyanide deaths support this view. Indeed, there is considerable variation in accounts. While reliability is not an issue, the question most raised relates to the method's 'peacefulness.' Just how peaceful is it to die with cyanide?

Most accounts of death from cyanide poisoning come from witnesses to gas chamber executions where the (unwilling) prisoner inhaled HCN. One study undertaken at San Quentin prison showed that, on average, consciousness was lost within one to three minutes, with death occurring after nine minutes. These deaths were often peaceful with the prisoner falling quickly asleep.

On some occasions, however, a violent (and presumably painful) death was observed. This method of execution was largely abandoned in the US in 1994 when the American Civil Liberties Union took a successful action against the California Department of Corrections. In their action, the ACLU argued successfully that the gas chamber violated the US Constitution's ban against cruel and unusual punishment, because it inflicted needless pain and suffering.

Eyewitness accounts of seriously ill people drinking dissolved cyanide salt are also mixed. In his book *Final Exit,* Derek Humphry describes deaths that are quick and painless. But he also documents one disturbing account that refers to a death that was 'miserable and violent, marked by frequent tetanic convulsions while awake' (Humphry, 1996: 30).

Toxicology texts of death by cyanide commonly refer to a rapid collapse and loss of consciousness if a large enough dose is absorbed. In his book *Suicide and Attempted Suicide: Methods and Consequences,* Geo Stone makes the observation that while cyanide might be commonly used by suicidal chemists, it is rarely by physicians. He concludes that this may be due to their different levels of access to poisons (Stone, 1999).

In 1995 when the guidelines for the *Northern Territory Rights of the Terminally Ill Act* (ROTI) were being developed the use of cyanide was not considered; better drugs (the barbiturates) were available. Nor is cyanide used in Oregon or Holland where euthanasia legislation is now in place. In *Final Exit* Humphrey summarises his thoughts on the use of cyanide, 'I believe that the balance of evidence about using cyanide indicates that it is best not used' (Humphry, 1996: 33).

The Availability of Cyanide

Soluble cyanide salts are generally hard to obtain unless one has a contact in the industries where these substances are used. These salts are also heavily regulated and restricted. They can however be manufactured (with care) from readily available ingredients, using unsophisticated facilities and equipment. Care must be employed in the manufacture, and the substance produced should be assayed to ensure the desired result.

The Manufacture of Sodium Cyanide

Sodium cyanide can be manufactured in a number of ways. Two relatively simple methods are described in the scientific literature. The first involves the use of the readily available dye, Prussian Blue (Iron III Ferro cyanide). A second uses the common swimming pool chlorine stabiliser, cyanuric acid.

In the first process the Prussian Blue is first converted to sodium ferrocyanide. This is done by allowing it to react with caustic soda in water. Iron oxide is precipitated and sodium ferro cyanide obtained. This sodium ferrocyanide (Yellow Prussate of Soda) is then converted to sodium cyanide by allowing it to react with concentrated sulphuric acid.

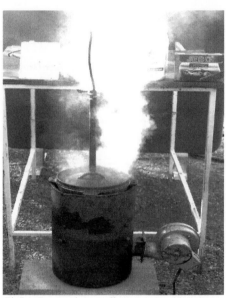

Fig7.1: Forge reduces sodium cyanate with carbon

The very toxic HCN produced is passed into caustic soda to form the desired salt. There is considerable information available on this process but it was abandoned after initial experiments, considering it too dangerous for the inexperienced home chemist - some of whom may be readers of this book.

A more suitable method of safe, small-scale home manufacture of sodium cyanide involves the two stage conversion of the common swimming pool chemical cyanuric acid.

The first step is carried out by heating powdered cyanuric acid with sodium carbonate. Sodium carbonate is obtained directly as washing soda (or by converting sodium bicarbonate, baking soda). In the second stage, the sodium cyanate produced is reduced to sodium cyanide by heating it with powdered charcoal in a covered crucible (Fig 7.1).

It is important that this stage is undertaken outside. In this process, carbon monoxide is given off. The resultant glassy mass is cooled, crushed and filtered with water to remove the soluble sodium cyanide from the remaining insoluble carbon (Fig 7.2). Careful drying produces solid sodium cyanide powder.

As with all home manufacture there is a need for great care in carrying out this process. Contaminated items need to be disposed of carefully after traces of cyanide are removed. This is best achieved using chlorine bleach to oxidise any unwanted cyanide and to prevent it contaminating the equipment. The product also needs to be tested by analytic means to determine its concentration and purity. Quantitative tests are available and Exit offers such a service for supporters. Further information that details the manufacturing process can be found in most university and public libraries.

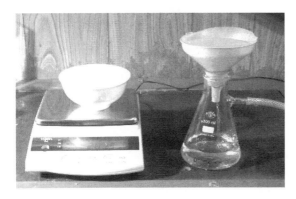

Fig 7.2: Filtering and weighing the sodium cyanide

Cyanide - RP Test

For a substance or drug to be useful as a Peaceful Pill two main criteria must be met. It must be, Reliable, and it must be Peaceful. Applying the Exit RP test to a salt like sodium cyanide gives some encouragement.

Reliability is high, few people will ever survive the ingestion of a sufficiently high dose of sodium cyanide. For a dose of 1gm of sodium cyanide, R=10.

There is also a correlation between the size of the dose and the speed of death and this minimises the chance of any adverse symptoms developing.

In terms of Peacefulness, the mixed accounts make this a difficult characteristic to assess. Clearly the size of the dose matters, if one is to minimise symptoms. Preparation is also important. The toxic effect is produced when stomach acid acts on the salt producing HCN which is then absorbed by the gut into the blood stream. This process is facilitated by dissolving the salt in cold water and drinking on an empty stomach where the gastric acid content is high.

An alternative is to place the cyanide salt into a treated gelatin capsule. Taking a 500mg capsule with an acidic drink (lemon juice, vinegar) creates the optimum conditions in the stomach. The delay can also usefully be employed to induce sleep with the addition of a strong soporific (sleeping tablet).

Taken in this manner the likelihood of a peaceful cyanide death is increased significantly. (P= 5)

Looking at the Minor Criteria:

Availability (2/5) - Soluble cyanide salts are generally hard to obtain unless one has a contact in the industries where these substances are used. These salts are heavily regulated and restricted. They can however be manufactured (with care) from readily available ingredients, using unsophisticated facilities and equipment. Care must be employed in the manufacture, and the substance produced should be assayed to ensure the desired result.

Preparation (5/5) - Cyanide salts are consumed as a drink or in a gelatin capsule. Some clinicians will note the pink colour and a possible smell of bitter almonds but this can often be missed, especially in cases where there is underlying serious illness.

Undetectability (3/5) - at autopsy the substance will be detected.

Speed (5/5) - optimal administration will cause a very quick death.

Safety (3/5) - there is little risk to others, although the glass should be washed. Note - if vomiting occurs, the gastric contents may give off dangerous HCN.

Storage (5/5). With proper storage, the sodium and potassium soluble cyanide salts have an almost indefinite shelf life.

Exit RP Score for Sodium Cyanide 38 (76%)

Exit RP Test

Criteria	Score
Reliability	*10/10*
Peacefulness	*5/10*
Availability	*2/5*
Preparation	*5/5*
Undetectability	*3/5*
Speed	*5/5*
Safety	*3/5*
Storage	*5/5*
Total	*38 (76%)*

Chapter 7: Frequently Asked Questions

- *Can one inhale the hydrogen cyanide gas rather than drinking the dissolved cyanide salt.?*

Yes, this can be very effective.

The process mimics that used in the US gas chamber where the solid cyanide salt (sodium, potassium or calcium cyanide) is added to concentrate acid. If 500ml of concentrated hydrochloric acid is placed in a plastic bucket and a few grams of the solid salt added there is a rapid production of hydrogen cyanide. If this is done in a confined space (a vehicle,or small room with windows shut) inhaling this gas leads to rapid and inevitable death. Concentrated hydrochloric acid (>25%) is readily available from hardware stores where it is marketed as a toilet cleaning agent, brick or paving cleaner, soldering flux or an agent for reducing the pH of a swimming pool.

The smell is sometimes reported as similar to that of bitter almonds, although some people, because of their genetic makeup, are unable to smell the gas. Be aware that the production of the gas may continue for some time and anyone entering the area may be unaware of the presence of the lethal gas. Warning signs must be posted to protect those who may come across the site. Safety on the Exit RP Test, is therefore low for this method 1/5 (see Carbon Monoxide, Ch6 and Hydrogen Sulfide, Ch8.).

8

Detergent Death

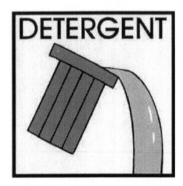 Since 2009, Exit has received requested for information on the so-called 'Detergent Suicide' method of ending one's life. While answers were provided to those asking the questions, it was not thought necessary to include details of the method in *The Peaceful Pill Handbook*.

This decision has been reviewed in 2011 and this chapter included. We stress however that the method scores poorly on the Exit RP test, and has little to recommend it. It is in effect a cheap and nasty suicide strategy, and readers are advised to consider other better alternatives outlined in this book.

The Method

The method makes use of the toxic nature of the gas hydrogen sulfide (H_2S) and it's ease of generation from readily available (unrestricted) household chemicals. Hydrogen Sulfide (commonly known as 'rotten egg gas') is extremely toxic when inhaled. The mechanism of action is similar to that of hydrogen cyanide (Chapter 7) where the gas binds with and destroys the function of mitochondria within living cells. The gas is as toxic as hydrogen cyanide, but accidental exposure is uncommon because of the strong and unpleasant smell noted with even the smallest concentrations of the gas.

Concentrations of over 0.1% (1000ppm) will lead to immediate loss of consciousness and rapid death. Production of the gas in a confined space (with levels in excess of 1%) will cause certain death.

Production of the Gas

The gas is easily produced using readily available ingredients. The usual method employed is to add a concentrated acid to an inorganic sulfide. For example adding concentrated hydrochloric acid to calcium sulfide leads to the rapid production of the gas.

$$2HCl + CaS \rightarrow H_2S + CaCl$$

The sulfide used in the early spate of Japanese suicides was reported as 'bath sulphur' a product used as a supplement added to bath water for therapeutic use. In western countries where there is little interest in sulphur baths, the commonest source of sulfides is the readily available 'Lime Sulphur' used as a common fungicide and insecticide by home gardeners. The major ingredient is calcium polysulfide (CaS_x) in aqueous solution.

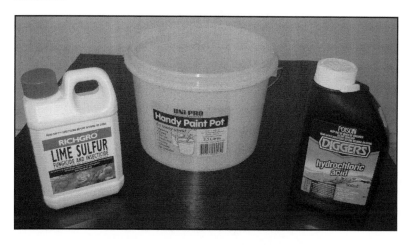

Fig 8.1 Simple ingredients used in Detergent Suicide

The addition of a strong acid to Lime Sulphur liquid in a plastic bucket results in the copious production of hydrogen sulfide gas. Common acids that release the gas include hydrochloric acid (HCl) available from hardware stores, and used as a paving, brick or toilet bowl cleaner, or as a swimming pool chemical, where it is used to lower the pH of the pool. An alternative acid that can be used in sulphuric acid (H_2SO_4) (See Chapter 6) which is used in vehicle lead acid batteries.

Problems with the method

While the ingredients required to make the gas are readily obtained, and unrestricted, the use of the gas to end one's life presents a number of significant problems. Of major concern is the risk to others when large amounts of hydrogen sulfide gas are produced. Apart from the likelihood of annoying everyone in the area with the stink, there are real dangers to those who might try to enter the area or attempt resuscitation. Indeed emergency personnel are trained to be careful entering an area where this gas is suspected, and not to attempt mouth to mouth resuscitation.

Clearly if one is planning to use this method it is essential that a site is chosen where leakage of the gas can not endanger innocent people and prominent warning signs should be displayed. The use of a car parked in an outdoor location with warning signs displayed prominently on the windows would seem to be the most responsible choice.

While it has been reported that as the concentration of the gas rises,there is a rapid inhibition of the sense of smell, so that one does not necessarily experience the sickening stench right to the point of death, it could not be considered a particularly peaceful.

The Exit RP Test

The method scores poorly for Peacefulness (P=2), but high on Reliability (R=10).

Considering the minor criteria: Availability & Speed score well at 5/5, Preparation & Storage at 4/5. However on Safety and Detectability, only the lowest score would be appropriate, giving a total score of only 30 (60%). The method therefore scores only slightly better than hanging (28, 56%), and less than the inhalation of carbon monoxide (31, 62%) (Chapter 4).

Exit RP Test

Criteria	Score
Reliability	*10/10*
Peacefulness	*2/10*
Availability	*5/5*
Preparation	*4/5*
Undetectability	*0/5*
Speed	*5/5*
Safety	*0/5*
Storage	*4/5*
Total	*30 (60%)*

9

Introduction to Drugs

Introduction

For many seriously ill people, taking drugs or substances orally (by mouth) is the preferred way to end life. Substances taken in this way (eg. Nembutal liquid) require no special equipment. It is this simplicity that explains the appeal of this version of the Peaceful Pill. The lack of any necessary bedside equipment also means that the death is more likely to be understood as one from 'natural causes'.

For example, if a person dying of cancer takes the final step by drinking Nembutal they will look as if they have died in their sleep. Most examining doctors would sign the death certificate indicating that this was the natural, expected death from their cancer. Of course, if an autopsy is undertaken, the causative drug will be discovered, but autopsies are increasingly rare in situations where the attending doctor believes the cause of death is clear (see Chapter 18).

However, while taking oral drugs might seem to be the simplest way of obtaining a peaceful and dignified death, the method does require planning. Knowledge of the substance to be used, its acquisition, preparation and administration are important.

The Role of the Drug Overdose

Generally speaking, drugs are developed to provide a cure to an illness or to give relief from symptoms. *Drugs are never developed to end life, at least not in humans.* Yet some drugs do cause death, especially if they are administered in ways that were never intended. The usual way to misuse a drug is to exceed the suggested dose: 'the overdose'.

While most drugs have side-effects (effects other than the purpose for which they are designed), and most side-effects are more pronounced when a drug is misused or taken in overdose, a side-effect like death is always going to be a serious problem for a drug manufacturer.

The company responsible for manufacturing a drug that will cause death in overdose will always be nervous about such a product and there will be a search to develop safer alternatives. So, while there are some drugs that do reliably cause death if misused, this number is small and decreasing. This process of replacing potentially lethal drugs with safer modern alternatives goes on all the time. The lethal barbiturates of earlier years have now been replaced by modern, safer sleeping tablets.

The lethal tri-cyclic antidepressants have almost disappeared, replaced by much safer serotonin uptake inhibitors like Prozac. Pain-relieving drugs like propoxyphene are currently under review and have already been replaced in many countries. The number of drugs that are of practical assistance to a seriously ill person seeking a peaceful death decreases each year.

Drugs, Swallowing and Taste

A person seeking a peaceful death will need to consume a lethal quantity of their chosen drug. These drugs are often bitter to taste, and consuming a large number of tablets can also be difficult if the person is suffering from a disease that effects swallowing. Examples include some diseases of the throat and oesophagus, or a disease like Motor Neurone Disease that can effect the muscles needed for swallowing. In some cases, problems with swallowing can be so severe that oral ingestion of drugs is simply not an option.

To avoid the bitter taste of the lethal dose, drugs are sometimes mixed with another substance to disguise the taste. Another approach is to spray the tongue and throat with a topical anaesthetic like Lignocaine. In Exit's experience neither of these strategies is particularly rewarding. This is because the drugs are often so bitter that mixing the drug with another substance, like yogurt or jam, simply creates a much larger quantity of an equally-unpleasant substance that then needs to be consumed. Anaesthetic sprays can work, but they are prescription items and require some expertise in administration.

The most effective method of consuming quantities of bitter-tasting drugs is to turn them into a liquid which can then be quickly drunk. This can be done by reducing tablets to powder with a mortar and pestle. Another way is to remove the gelatin covering of the capsules and dissolving the powder in a common solvent such as water. Even if a drug does not fully dissolve, a fine powder can still be made drinkable by rapid stirring with a teaspoon. A suspension of fine particles can usually be swallowed without much difficulty.

By keeping the volume of the liquid to be drunk to 100ml (approx. 1/3 cup), only a few mouthfuls are needed. The bitter after-taste is effectively dealt with by following this drink with another stronger tasting drink - usually alcohol (see Drugs & Alcohol).

Drugs and Vomiting

Any substance taken orally can be vomited up, and concern about this can cause considerable anxiety. A person intending to die must take the full (lethal) amount, so it is important to ensure that vomiting does not occur. Some people are prone to vomiting, and some diseases can cause vomiting. In a minority of cases vomiting, or fear of vomiting, can be such a problem that it is not possible to use oral drugs.

To minimize the risk of vomiting, an anti-vomiting ('anti-emetic') drug is usually taken for a period of time before the consumption of the lethal drug. There are a number of drugs used for this purpose.

Anti-emetics are readily obtained, although the most effective are prescription items. The most common are metoclopramide (Maxolon, Pramin, Paspertin) and prochlorperazine (Stemetil, Stemazine). One common procedure is to take six tablets (ie 60mg metoclopramide as a 'stat' dose) about 40 minutes before taking the lethal drug. Another procedure is to take the anti-emetic for a full two days before the lethal drug is to be consumed (here the usual dose is two tablets every 8 hours). With this method there is then no need to synchronise the time at which the anti-vomiting drugs are taken with the taking of the lethal drugs.

If anti-vomiting drugs are taken, the risk of vomiting is very low and problems are rare, except in cases where vomiting is a known specific problem. In these cases alternative methods should be explored.

Unless there are specific questions of hypersensitivity or allergy (which are very unusual), the anti-emetic 'Maxolon' is recommended. The dose (60mg stat or 20mg 3x/day for 2 days) is independent of the quantity of the lethal drug.

If vomiting does occur, the individual should bring up (vomit up) as much of the drug from their stomach as they can and the attempt to end their life should be abandoned. Ipecac Syrup can be used to encourage vomiting. It is advisable to have some on hand and can be obtained from the local pharmacy.

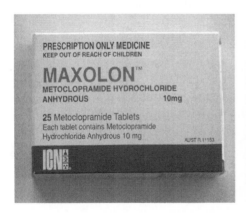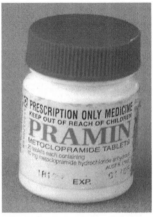

Fig 9.1: The common antiemetic metoclopramide

Drugs & Alcohol

Alcohol is often used as a supplement when drugs are used to end life. It serves several functions. Firstly, lethal drugs taken orally are often bitter and leave a prolonged unpleasant after-taste. Even when the drug is consumed in a few quick mouthfuls, a seriously ill person can find this taste quite distressing. Strong alcohol is effective in removing this after-taste. As this is to be the person's last drink a favoured spirit or liqueur is often chosen. People sip at their favourite Scotch or Baileys Irish Cream and the bitter taste quickly disappears.

Secondly, alcohol plays a useful role in 'potentiating' the lethal drug. To follow the drug with an alcoholic drink will usually enhance its speed of action and potency. This is true of most of the commonly-used lethal, oral drugs.

Thirdly, alcohol is a useful calming agent (anxiolytic) in what is inevitably a stressful time. It is important that any alcohol is taken *after* the consumption of the lethal drugs so that there is no clouding of a person's mind.

Note though, people should not force themselves to drink alcohol, especially if they find the thought distasteful. The drugs described in this book cause death, with or without alcohol. The most likely effect of excluding the alcohol is that the process will take longer. Liquid morphine (Ordine) can be used as a supplement/potentiator by people with an aversion to alcohol.

Drug Tolerance

Exposure to a particular drug over a prolonged period of time can often lead to the development of an insensitivity to that drug. If a drug is being taken for a particular medical purpose (eg. the relief of pain), one might find that after a while the same pain relief can only be obtained by increasing the dose. This is known as 'tolerance.'

Some drugs are particularly prone to this effect. The body's response to opiates like morphine or pethidine is an example. After taking morphine for even a short time, the effect of a particular dose will lessen and greater amounts will be needed to achieve the same pain-relieving effect.

After a period off the drugs, one's sensitivity usually returns. This explains why people often accidentally die when taking illegal narcotics like heroin. A person who regularly uses heroin soon develops a tolerance for it. If they are unable to continue taking the drug - perhaps because their supply has broken down or perhaps they have spent time in an institution, they will redevelop their sensitivity. When a new supply becomes available, their greater sensitivity increases the likelihood of accidental death (see Chapter 10 for more information on the opiates).

Tolerance to a particular drug can be an important factor when choosing a drug to end one's life. If a seriously ill person has been taking a drug for some time and has developed a tolerance for this particular drug, the necessary 'lethal dose' for the drug can be higher than that usually quoted.

Slow Release (SR) and Enteric Coated (EC) Drugs

Some drugs are treated in some way so as to effect the rate or manner in which they are absorbed into the human body. Examples include 'Slow release' and 'Enteric Coated' forms of the pharmaceutical.

Drugs packaged in a way that allows a slow, steady absorption from the gut into the blood stream are called 'Slow release' and often given the initials 'SR'. Some of the drugs are used to provide a peaceful death are available in SR forms, but one should be aware that these forms of the drug are usually *less effective than standard preparations.*

This is because the drug's lethal effect usually depends on a rapid rise in the level of the drug in a person's blood (ie. at a rate that is too fast for the body's normal excretion mechanisms). Slow Release forms *do not* cause a steep rise in the blood level of the drug. Crushing or dissolving the drugs before consumption is unlikely to alter this. *Powdered, slow release drugs are still slow release.* Morphine (NOT the best end of life drug - see Chapter 10) is often prescribed in slow release tablet forms to ensure long periods of pain control, and is less effective in this form.

Enteric Coating, is a way of treating some pharmaceuticals so that the active ingredient passes to a more receptive part of the gut before being absorbed into the bloodstream. Examples include those drugs that may be partially destroyed by the strong acid environment of the stomach, but are stable, potent and readily absorbed in the alkaline duodenum and upper small intestine. Enteric coatings inevitably slow the release of active pharmaceuticals and are best avoided. Some anti-emetic (anti vomiting) drugs come in EC forms.

Alternative Routes of Administration of Drugs

Stomach PEGs & Nasogastric (NG) Tubes

People who have difficulty swallowing sometimes have a surgical procedure that allows the introduction of liquid food directly into the stomach. This feeding tube is inserted through the wall of the abdomen and is called a percutaneous endoscopic gastrostomy (PEG tube) 'stomach peg'.

The administration of drugs is often easier for a person who has a peg. There are no concerns over bitter taste, vomiting, or the person's ability to swallow the required quantity of the drug. For a person with a PEG, a drug can be injected directly into the stomach.

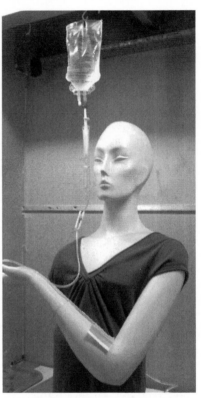

Nasogastric tubes are also occasionally used to provide fluids to someone who is having difficulty swallowing. This temporary procedure sees a small diameter tube positioned through the nose and down the throat into the stomach. It is possible to deliver fluids directly into the stomach through such a tube.

Fig 9.2: Intravenous drug administration

Lethal drugs given in this way need to be in liquid form.

Intravenous Drugs

Many drugs are delivered directly into the body through a needle or cannula that is placed into a vein. Drugs delivered by this route must be liquids. The procedure of inserting a needle into a vein requires a degree of expertise and this can be difficult for people who have not had some medical or nursing training.

The speed of action of any drug administered in this way is much greater than for those administered orally. The rapid effect of such administration can occasionally cause difficulty. If the person decides to inject the drug themselves they may loose consciousness before the required dose has been delivered.

To ensure that the full lethal dose is administered intravenously, a bag of saline can be used. The saline bag is attached to a cannula through a standard intravenous 'giving set' (Fig 9.2). The drugs are added to the saline and continue to flow, even if consciousness is lost, although there is always the risk that the intravenous access will be lost if the cannula is mechanically dislodged.

One advantage of intravenous administration is that it extends the range of drugs that can be used. Some drugs that are not well absorbed through the gut when taken orally, drugs like potassium, can cause death when administered intravenously.

Rectal Administration

Drugs are occasionally administered rectally using suppositories, or by direct infusion (enema). This is usually done if there is difficulty swallowing or if vomiting is a problem. Some lethal drugs can be quickly absorbed in this way, and occasionally this provides a way of proceeding if there are intractable difficulties associated with oral administration.

Resuscitation

The act of taking a lethal drug does not result in an immediate death. Rather, the time that elapses from consuming the drugs until death, depends on a number of factors, and this time can occasionally lead to failure.

Some drugs or substances taken orally act very quickly. In some cases, speed of death *is* an important factor, such as the case of a spy taking a suicide pill to prevent interrogation or torture. For example, Hermann Goering used cyanide in his cell the night before he was due to be executed. Although Goering was being watched very closely, his death was so quick that resuscitation was impossible. However, such a rapid death is rarely a consideration for a seriously ill person wanting to put an end to their suffering.

People often think of a 'peaceful death' as dying in one's sleep, and drugs that cause this are sought out. The time spent asleep before death can vary considerably. The longer this time, the greater the likelihood of some unexpected intervention. To reduce any chance of this, it is in the person's interest to obtain those drugs which bring about sleep, loss of consciousness, then death, relatively quickly. This is one clear advantage of the barbiturate, Nembutal where sleep occurs within minutes of consumption of the drug and alcohol, with death following usually within the hour.

Other commonly-used drugs have a much longer 'window period' when intervention can occur. For the common propoxyphene/oxazepam combination (see Chapter 11), this window period may be a matter of hours. This means that considerable planning may be needed to reduce the chance of discovery during this time.

The possibility of unwanted intervention is why many people prefer to take lethal drugs in the evening when there is an expected period of several hours before any chance of discovery. If the deeply unconscious person were to be found before death, this can present a significant problem to the person tasked with, or who accidentally, finds them. Even if they are aware of the unconscious person's plan, the discoverer must do something to protect themselves. It would not be acceptable, for example, to claim in the morning that you noticed that your friend or partner was unconscious but you chose to do nothing about it. During the night a person might argue that they had been asleep and hadn't noticed, but in the morning, the situation changes. A person in this position needs to consider their options carefully.

If an ambulance is called, the discoverer will be protected, but the attending paramedics will attempt to resuscitate the unconscious person and this may well thwart their wish to die. Remember, ambulance paramedics are generally under no legal obligation to abide by a person's Advance Medical Directive (AMD) (Living Will/ Do Not Resuscitate (DNR) notice). The Officers attending will usually say that these issues 'can be sorted out at the hospital.' (For more discussion about the pros and cons of AMDs and role of emergency workers see my first book - *Killing Me Softly: Voluntary Euthanasia and the Road to the Peaceful Pill.*)

Alternatively, someone discovering an unconscious person may protect themselves by calling the family physician. The physician should be aware if a AMD exists and can avoid initiating resuscitation without risking legal repercussions. A doctor who knows the background may well begin a morphine infusion ("to make the patient comfortable"), and allow their patient to peacefully die.

The Shelf Life of Drugs

Most drugs are subject to some form of degradation over time. This may be brought about by chemical, physical or microbial breakdown. The main impact of degradation on a drug is the loss of potency.

To ensure that drugs are as effective as possible, manufacturers include storage instructions and an 'expiry date' with each item. The time taken from manufacture to expiry date is referred to as the drug's 'shelf life' and it is in the manufacturers' interest to make this as long as possible. Clearly a drug will not be rendered ineffective after the stated expiry date. Rather, this date merely indicates that if stored correctly, no significant chemical, physical or microbial degradation of the drug will have occurred before this date.

Research shows that many drugs remain highly effective for many years after their expiry date. For modern medicines, expiration dates are usually set for two to three years after the date of the manufacture of the drug. This is the case for veterinary liquid Nembutal which has a shelf life/ expiry date stamped on the side of the bottle, but has been shown to be very effective for many years after this date.

Also, the form of the drug will often effect its shelf life. For example, pills and capsules stored in their original, air-tight containers at cool room temperatures and free from humidity are often viable for around 10 years. This is much longer than the stated expiry date. The powdered form of a drug (eg. Chinese powder Nembutal) has similar longevity, especially if it is vacuum-packed (using a standard kitchen food vacuum-sealer) and kept cool and away from light. For drugs in liquid form, the shelf life is commonly shorter.

To tell if a drug has deteriorated, there are some common sense guidelines.

In the case of a liquid, the drug's appearance is important. One should check its colour and clarity (has it become cloudy); particulate matter (eg. are there tiny visible particles); preservative content (if stated); sterility (has the bottle been tampered with or opened) and whether the drug has interacted with its enclosure (bottle or lid). If none of these signs are present, then the liquid in question is more likely to be viable, than if there were any signs of degradation.

If the drug is in tablet form, signs of degradation include the tablet's appearance, moisture content, hardness (have the tablets become as hard as rocks), friability (uncoated tablets), disintegration time (when placed in water) and uniformity of content. Again, any of these tell-tale signs may indicate chemical degradation.

Of course, the only certain way of establishing whether significant degradation has taken place is by carrying out a chemical assay on the product. For drugs that are hard to obtain and difficult to replace with fresh samples, an assay makes a lot of sense. A detailed discussion on the testing of the purity and potency of Nembutal is given in Chapter 15.

To tell if a drug has deteriorated, there are some common sense guidelines.

In the case of a liquid, the drug's appearance is important. One should check its colour and clarity (has it become cloudy); particulate matter (eg. are there tiny visible particles); preservative content (if stated); sterility (has the bottle been tampered with or opened) and whether the drug has interacted with its enclosure (bottle or lid). If none of these signs are present, then the liquid in question is more likely to be viable, than if there were any signs of degradation.

If the drug is in tablet form, signs of degradation include the tablet's appearance, moisture content, hardness (have the tablets become as hard as rocks), friability (uncoated tablets), disintegration time (when placed in water) and uniformity of content. Again, any of these tell-tale signs may indicate chemical degradation.

Of course, the only certain way of establishing whether significant degradation has taken place is by carrying out a chemical assay on the product. For drugs that are hard to obtain and difficult to replace with fresh samples, an assay makes a lot of sense. A detailed discussion on the testing of the purity and potency of Nembutal is given in Chapter 15.

Conclusion

This Chapter details some of the most important issues that should be considered if a person is planning to use drugs to achieve a peaceful, dignified death.

Specific issues such as preparation, administration, vomiting, and the shelf-life of a drug are common to all drugs, and an understanding of these issues reduces the chance of failure. This Chapter should be read in conjunction with the chapters that detail the use of particular drugs (Chapters 10 - 15).

10

Drug Options - Morphine
&
Slow Euthanasia

Introduction - The Doctor's Loophole

Slow euthanasia or the 'Doctrine of Double Effect' as it is often called, is the only way a caring doctor can hasten the death of a patient and escape any legal consequence.

Known commonly as the 'doctor's loophole' slow euthanasia allows a doctor to end a patient's life by slowly increasing the amount of a pain-killing drug. In the eyes of the law it doesn't matter if, in the course of treating a person's pain, the person dies.

It is the administration of the pain-relieving drug that causes the double effect; it relieves pain but it also causes death. As long as the stated primary intention is the treatment of the person's pain, the doctor is legally safeguarded.

While slow euthanasia is relatively common, few doctors will ever admit their involvement. Even while administering slow euthanasia, some doctors will argue that they are only treating the patient's pain. Others know exactly what their 'prime intention' is, but wisely decide to keep quiet about it. Others just prefer not to think about it too closely.

It is a pity that this practice is so cloaked in secrecy. Clearly, it would be better if there were open and honest communication between the medical system (represented in the doctor and health care team), the patient and the patient's family. However, with laws in place that make it a serious crime to hasten a patient's death, but make it no crime at all to aggressively treat pain, there is little prospect of change.

How Slow Euthanasia Works in Practice

A doctor practising slow euthanasia usually gives a narcotic analgesic (morphine), while periodically reviewing the patient's pain. The claim is then made that treatment is inadequate, and the morphine dose increased.

If this review takes place every 4 - 6 hours, morphine levels will rise. Eventually lethal levels will be reached and the patient will die. The doctor defends his or her actions by simply saying that they were trying to control the patient's pain. Death, they argue, was an unplanned consequence of either the patient's disease or the necessary treatment for the pain.

It can take days for the levels of morphine to become high enough to cause death. It is important for the doctor's safety that the process is slow. Indeed, it is the length of time taken that gives credibility to the argument that there was effort put into establishing just the right dose of morphine.

Another way of understanding the process of slow euthanasia is to consider the link between cause and effect. The time taken for the morphine to end life muddies the water and blurs the connection between the cause (the commencement of morphine) and the effect (the patient's death). By blurring this link, a doctor can help a patient die and escape the legal consequences.

Problems with Slow Euthanasia

Slow euthanasia has a number of features that limit its appeal to a patient. Firstly, it is the doctor who is in control. While a patient might ask for this form of help, it will be the doctor who decides if and when it will be provided. Just because you - the patient - feel that now is the right time to begin the process, there is no guarantee that the doctor will agree.

They may feel you should wait; wait until you become sicker, perhaps until your haemoglobin drops a few points, or your respiratory function tests deteriorate further. The sicker you are, the safer it is for the doctor to go down this path. If the doctor disagrees with you and thinks the 'best time' to help should be several weeks away, there is absolutely nothing you can do about it.

Another drawback of slow euthanasia is the restriction on the range of drugs that a doctor might use to help a person die. If the doctor's defence is to be that it was the treatment of the patient's pain that caused the death, then a pain-relieving drug like morphine must be used.

A doctor could not, for example, administer a large dose of a barbiturate. While a barbiturate might provide the most peaceful and quickest death, barbiturates are not pain relieving drugs, and the claim that such a drug was being used to treat pain makes no sense.

This use of morphine by doctors to end life has led to the common community misconception that the best drug to use to end one's life is morphine - it must be, because that's the drug doctors use! This unfortunate misunderstanding leads to many failed suicide attempts.

And the process must be slow. Indeed, slow euthanasia can often take days or even weeks. Often the patient is given a sedative that keeps them asleep through the whole process; midazolam is the drug of choice.

Coupled with morphine, this morphine - midazolam mix (known as 'Double M Therapy') places the patient in an induced coma for the time needed to raise the morphine level sufficiently. Double M therapy allows the patient to sleep through their own death and gives rise to another name for the process - 'pharmacological oblivion.'

The doctor still makes the assessment about the need for larger and larger morphine doses. Here the decision is based not on the patient's complaints, but upon a clinical assessment of the unconscious person.

The doctor will also choose the place of death. It is unusual for slow euthanasia to take place in a patient's home. Usually it occurs in an institution, commonly a hospital or hospice.

In an institution, a team is often involved in providing care and several doctors might participate in the relentless increase of the morphine. This further blurs the link between cause and effect and makes it even safer for the medical staff involved. While slow euthanasia could take place at the patient's home, in practice this presents many logistical difficulties. The doctor would need to make many visits, perhaps several a day, to facilitate the relentless increase in drugs.

Also full nursing care is required; an unconscious patient needs to be moved regularly and watched constantly to ensure the flow of drugs is not interrupted. This is often an extremely difficult time for those close to the patient as they find themselves participating in this deliberate, slow death watch.

For these reasons, few people opt for slow euthanasia as their preferred choice for a peaceful, dignified death. More commonly, it is an option of desperation, when few alternatives exist. In such dire circumstances, if a doctor does offer help (usually through a nod, a wink and an understanding), patients will grab the chance, reasoning correctly, that this is better than nothing.

Those who are left often see this as an example of a doctor helping someone to die, and this leads to the commonly expressed view that there is no need for euthanasia legislation. People say 'I can't see what all the fuss is about with voluntary euthanasia – it goes on all the time – doctors are always helping people to die.'

It is as well to remember that 'what goes on all the time' is the grim process of suspending a sick person by a thread between life and death for an arbitrary time, until the thread breaks.

That is slow euthanasia!

Asking for Slow Euthanasia

The process of slow euthanasia is always controlled by the doctor. Because of this, there is usually little a patient can do to ensure that the option is available. Often when patients realize that they have a deteriorating medical condition, they ask their doctor whether or not they will be able to help them 'at the end.' The doctor may even volunteer to have this discussion and this is encouraging - but be careful.

When doctor and patient begin speaking in this tangential way, there is a very real chance that significant misunderstandings can occur. It is not uncommon for a doctor to promise 'every assistance when the time comes' and for the patient to draw immense comfort from this.

A patient might even imagine that the doctor is saying that 'when things deteriorate I will give you access to lethal drugs.' In reality, this is highly unlikely. Few medical doctors would risk de-registration and a significant jail term. The only assistance likely from the doctor, is for them to initiate slow euthanasia, with the patient being admitted to an institution, a hospital or hospice. And there may well be argument about when the process should commence.

Exit suggests that in situations where slow euthanasia has appeal, that early discussions between patient and doctor take place. Be blunt. If the doctor promises help 'when the time comes', insist on knowing who will decide when that time is, and exactly what sort of help is being promised?

If there is any attempt to skirt or dismiss your questions, be very wary. Try discussing the issue with another doctor, or look into an alternative end of life strategy.

The Role of Opiates and Opioids

Opiates are naturally occurring compounds that originate from the sap of the poppy, *papaver somniferum*. Substances derived from these compounds are opioids. These compounds all effect the same receptors in the brain and are generally used for the control of strong pain.

While morphine is the commonest example, other examples include, pethidine, codeine, methadone and fentanyl. The illegal drug heroin is also an opiate. All opiates have properties that make them difficult drugs for a person to use to reliably end their life.

The biggest problem associated with taking opiates is predicting the effect. There is remarkable individual variability in sensitivity to these drugs within the normal population. People who are similar physically (same height, weight, sex etc) can have a vastly different response to the administration of an opiate.

A small dose of morphine may have almost no effect on one person, while that same dose could kill another. Predicting the effect of the drug on an individual is difficult. When these drugs are used clinically the rule of thumb has been to 'start low and go slow' until the individual's sensitivity to the drug is established.

Another difficulty with opiates is the rapid development of tolerance when the drugs are taken for any period of time. Within days, the morphine that initially had a powerful effect on the pain can become almost ineffective.

To obtain the same pain relief the dose must be increased. If these drugs are taken for long periods, very large doses might be needed to provide adequate pain control. These required doses can become so large that if they were taken before the tolerance had developed, death could well have been the result.

It is this development of tolerance, and its rapid loss once the drugs stop, that often leads to the accidental death of people who self-administer opiates, especially heroin. If there is a break in supply and the acquired tolerance is lost, a sudden resumption may result in an unexpected fatal overdose.

Opioids

Natural
Opium
Morphine
Heroin
Codeine

Semi Synthetic
Heroin

Synthetic
Pethadine
Methadone
Fentanyl

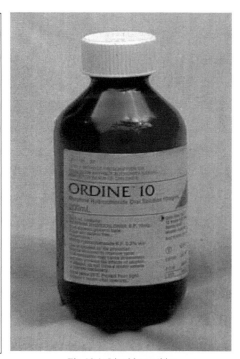

Fig 10.1: Liquid morphine

Morphine is commonly prescribed as a slow release (SR) tablet. MS Contin and Kapanol are marketed forms. These may be taken once or twice a day and slowly release the morphine to give 'background' pain control. For the onset of sudden (breakthrough) pain, a fast release form of the drug, liquid morphine is often prescribed (Ordine).

Many very sick people receive these drugs for the pain of serious illness and sometimes go to great lengths to stockpile tablets believing that they will soon acquire a lethal dose. But knowing how many morphine tablets to accumulate is like asking the length of a piece of string?

A single dose of SR tablet morphine may cause death, but the result is often unpredictable. The fast-acting liquid morphine may be a more effective form of the drug, but the problems of sensitivity and tolerance remain.

For these reasons it is difficult to advocate the opiates as stand-alone, single-dose, oral agents to provide a reliable death. One exception to this general rule is propoxyphene (see Chapter 11). When this drug is taken with a (non-lethal) benzodiazepine, a reliable death will occur.

The opiates do, however, have a role as supplementary or potentiating agents, (ie. a drug taken to enhance the effectiveness of another drug). This role is usually filled by alcohol, but for people who do not drink, morphine liquid can be a good alternative.

The Use of Heroin

Exit is occasionally asked about whether heroin should be obtained from 'the street' and used to end life. These questions are often prompted by news reports of people dying from a heroin overdose. In reality, there is little to be gained by using heroin.

As an opiate heroin suffers from the problems of tolerance and sensitivity mentioned above. In addition there is the question of the uncertainty of the dose with heroin. Because it has been acquired on the streets, one can never be exactly sure what or how much one has actually purchased. It also needs to be injected intravenously. In Exit's experience, few elderly and seriously ill people have these skills.

Note: If heroin is taken orally, it turns back into morphine in the gut and offers no advantage over prescription tablet morphine, where at least the exact dose is known.

One final point on the opiates. If one does die taking these drugs, the death is likely to be very peaceful. Morphia is, after all, the goddess of dreams.

Conclusion

In Exit's internal polling of over 1000 of our supporters, less than one percent (0.3%) of Exit members say that they would prefer slow euthanasia compared to a Peaceful Pill (89%). Slow euthanasia is, therefore, one of the least-preferred methods of dying, and one that is usually avoided when other options exist. Given a choice, people prefer to have control of the dying process.

This is not the case with slow euthanasia. It is relatively rare to find someone who wants to spend their last days in a drug-induced coma. When people decide that their suffering is so great that death is preferable, they want their passing to be quick.

This is why slow euthanasia is almost always an option of last resort. It is the method accepted when nothing else is on offer, and the only alternative is relentless and ongoing suffering.

Finally, there remains a common belief that the 'opiates' are the best drugs to end life. This undeserved reputation comes from their almost-universal use in slow euthanasia, where doctors have little choice.

While a single overdose of morphine *may* cause death, individual sensitivity and tolerance to these drugs make this an uncertain and unpredictable process. The opiates are best used to do the job they are designed to do, control strong pain. There are *better* euthanasia options available.

The Exit RP Test for Morphine

Morphine (or any of the other opiates) do not score particularly well on the RP Test. When used as a drug and taken as a single dose by a person wanting to die, the difficulty of establishing the lethal dose significantly reduces Reliability (4/10). Peacefulness though is good (10/10).

Minor criteria scores are patchy. Availability (3/5), sometimes morphine is available - if a person is suffering from a recognised painful disease. But the use of the opiates as drugs of addiction and their place in the illegal narcotic trade can also make them occasionally very difficult to obtain. Preparation is easy (5/5), although constricted 'pinpoint' pupils can often alert a medical officer to the presence of these drugs in the system (Undetectability = 2/5). Death can also take some time, depending on one's tolerance and resuscitation is often straightforward using the opiate antagonist Naloxone (Speed = 2/5). There are no safety issues (Safety = 5/5), and the drug has a moderate shelf life (Storage = 3/5).

Exit RP Test - Morphine

Criteria	Score
Reliability	*4/10*
Peacefulness	*10/10*
Availability	*3/5*
Preparation	*5/5*
Undetectability	*2/5*
Speed	*2/5*
Safety	*5/5*
Storage	*3/5*
Total	*34 (68%)*

11

Drug Options - Propoxyphene

Introduction

A useful, lethal drug, still prescribed in a handful of countries, is propoxyphene. The drug is marketed under various names and used as an oral analgesic (pain reliever). If prepared in a certain way, and taken in combination with a common benzodiazepine sleeping pill such as oxazepam (Serepax), propoxyphene will provide a reliable, peaceful and dignified death.

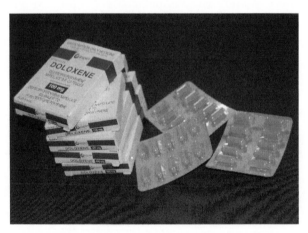

Fig 11.1
Propoxphene capsules (Doloxene)

The Various Forms of Propoxyphene

Propoxyphene is marketed under a number of names, examples include Darvon, Doloxene, and Depronal.

Regardless of its name, the key necessary ingredient is propoxyphene – either as the hydrochloride or napsylate, and it is important that the drug labels are read very carefully. In some video segments included in this chapter the name Doloxene is used to refer to propoxyphene.

Propoxyphene capsules have only one active ingredient (dextropropoxyphene napsylate). However, the drug propoxyphene is often marketed in combination with other common analgesics such as paracetemol (acetaminophen) and marketed as Di-Gesic (Darvocet).

These combination products are of limited use. Taking a large amount of the associated drug can complicate the process. The ingestion of a substantial quantity of paracetemol (acetominophen) for example may well lead to death, but it would not be regarded as particularly peaceful.

Note: With the withdrawal of the barbiturate sleeping tablets from the medical prescribing list, Doloxene has become the most common doctor-prescribed medication used by seriously ill people to end their lives. Recently, the unique properties of Doloxene have begun to attract attention; first in the UK, then New Zealand and more recently in the US and Canada where it has now been removed from the prescribing schedule. It is expected that Doloxene will soon be restricted or removed from the prescribing lists of many countries.

When is Propoxyphene Prescribed?

Propoxyphene (dextropropoxyphene napsylate) is almost always available from a doctor on prescription, where it is used for pain management. Propoxyphene is usually prescribed when over-the-counter pain relievers prove inadequate and when other, more common prescription pain-relievers (eg. Panadeine Forte or Tylenol-Codeine - a mixture of paracetemol and codeine) prove unsatisfactory.

Propoxyphene can be used whenever there is a need for general pain relief. Before their removal in late 2010 in the US (and Canada), propoxyphene and combinations were the 12th most prescribed generic drug (Public Citizen, 2006)

How Lethal is Propoxyphene?

Propoxyphene has a very narrow therapeutic margin. The difference in dose between that providing analgesia and that causing death is small. Like the opioids, the outcome from a particular dose can be difficult to predict (See Chapter 10), but this drug produces a cardio-toxic metabolite when it breaks down which increases its usefulness as a self deliverance agent.

When another drug, the readily-available, non-lethal sleeping tablet, oxazepam, is added, along with alcohol, the result is certain. Exit has no reported failures from this combination.

As the reputation of propoxyphene has grown, so script sizes have been reduced. The standard packaging number for propoxyphene is now 50 capsules. All capsules contain the same 100mg of dextropropoxyphene napsylate.

If 10gm of dextropropoxyphene napsylate powder is obtained from 100 capsules and taken with 10 or more moderately, long-acting sleeping tablets like oxazepam, death will follow.

Propoxyphene is usually prescribed at the rate of 4-6 capsules per day (400 - 600 mg) to deal with pain. Ten grams of the drug would provide around 2 to 3 weeks of pain control.

The Role of Oxazepam

Oxazepam (Serepax) is a moderately long-acting, non-lethal sleeping tablet. Another moderately long-acting sleeping tablet often used in combination with propoxyphene is nitrazepam (Mogadon). These modern sleeping tablets are members of a drug class known as benzodiazepines and when taken by themselves are not usually lethal, even if taken in large amounts. When taken in combination with propoxyphene, oxazepam or nitrazepam reinforce the effect of a propoxyphene and a lethal combination is the result.

Note: Duration of action of the benzodiazepine is important - shorter acting drugs like temazepam are not recommended.

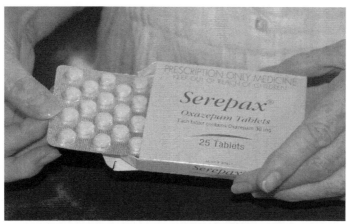

Fig 11.2: The common sleeping tablet - oxazepam (Serapax)

When is Oxazepam Prescribed?

Well known as sleeping drugs, oxazepam and nitrazepam are available on prescription from a doctor. They are prescribed for insomnia (when a person is unable to sleep). Oxazepam is usually prescribed in packets containing 25 sleeping tablets, which come in two sizes, 15mg and 30mg.

People using propoxyphene, often take a full packet of 30mg oxazepam tablets as the supplement.

Taking Propoxyphene

The drugs are taken sequentially. Prepare the propoxyphene by pulling apart 100 x 100mg capsules (or cut them open with scissors) and empty the 10gm white dextropropoxyphine napsylate powder into a glass. In another glass place 10 or more 30mg oxazepam tablets and cover them with water.

It is wise to take an anti-emetic (eg metoclopramide) either as a single stat dose or for 48 hours before the planned death (see Chapter 9). After having something light to eat, add enough water to the 10gm of propoxyphine powder so that stirring allows the drug to be drunk. Note: the napsylate does not dissolve in the water, stir with a spoon and then drink the suspension of particles. Stir the second glass with the oxazepam and water till this also can be taken as a drink.

Alcohol is useful to take away the bitter drug after-taste and will speed the process. Sit comfortably. In 10 - 20 minutes sleep will occur and death will follow usually in 4 - 6 hours.

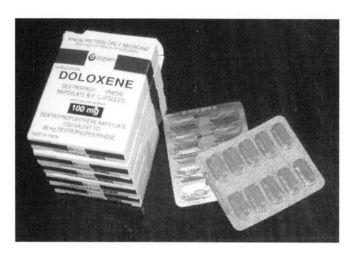

Fig 11.3
100mg pink Doloxene Capsules

Shelf Life of Doloxene

Propoxyphene has a relatively long shelf life. Prescribed capsules have an expiry date stamped on each card and this is usually 2 or 3 years into the future. Although this provides only a rough guide, in the absence of any available testing of the drug, it is the only indication one has. Capsules that have reached their expiry date should be treated with caution (See Chapter 8 for a discussion on shelf life).

The Future of Propoxyphene

Propoxyphene faces an uncertain future. The withdrawal of the drug from the prescription schedule in the UK in early 2005. The drug has also been withdrawn in the European Union, the US, Canada and in New Zealand. In November 2010 the FDA announced that the drug would be also removed from the US market.
http://nyti.ms/9iPzgD

At the time of press, propoxyphene is still available on prescription in Australia, Mexico and a range of South American and Asian countries.

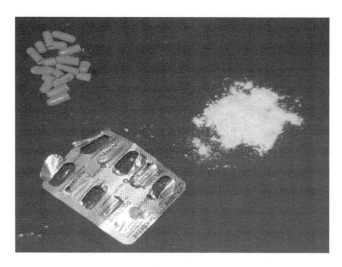

Fig 11.4: Propoxyphene powder ready for mixing with water

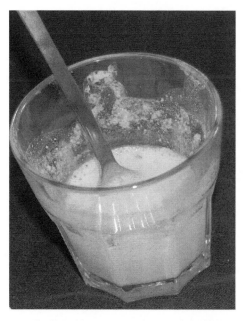

Fig 11.5: 10gm propoxyphene ready to drink

RP Test for Propoxyphene

Propoxyphene scores well on the RP Test. Exit has no confirmed reports of failure and it rates 9/10 for Reliability. The time before sleep occurs is longer than other drugs like Nembutal and this can cause anxiety. Peacefulness (7/10).

In the minor categories: Availability is listed at 4/5. Most people who set out to get this drug will acquire it. Remember though that if the drug is withdrawn, availability will drop to zero. Preparation is more complicated than with other ingestibles (Pr=3/5). The drug is undetectable - unless there is an autopsy, although constricted pupils may cause suspicion (D=3/5). The process is slow (Sp=2/5) the drug presents no risk to others (Sa=5/5). The drug has a moderate shelf life (St=3/5). Total 36 or 72%

RP Test for Propoxyphene

Criteria	Score
Reliability	**9/10**
Peacefulness	**7/10**
Availability	**4/5**
Preparation	**3/5**
Undetectability	**3/5**
Speed	**2/5**
Safety	**5/5**
Storage	**3/5**
Total	**36 (72%)**

12

Other Drugs and Common Myths

In this chapter a number of other drug options for a peaceful death are considered. Although sometimes thought of as reliably lethal, each of these possible pharmeceutical options suffers from some factor or issue that makes the choice less desirable than the gold standard, Nembutal.

The drugs to be considered in this chapter include:

• The tricyclic antidepressant - Amitriptyline
• The hormone - Insulin

Amitriptyline

Amitriptyline is the most useful in a class of drugs known as tricyclic antidepressants (TCAs). These drugs can be lethal if taken in a certain way.

The TCAs date back to the early 1960s where they established themselves as useful antidepressants. However, their narrow therapeutic margin (the dose needed for therapy as an antidepressant and that which is toxic is close) meant that there were dangers in prescribing these drugs, especially to depressed people, from either accidental or intentional overdose.

Their implication in a large number of deaths from overdose meant that other classes of safer antidepressants such as the seratonin re-uptake inhibitors (SSRI) like fluoxetine (Prozac) found favour and largely displaced the TCAs.

Since this time the TCAs have undergone something of a resurgence for the treatment of intractable neuropathic pain (such as trigeminal neuralgia) and migraine.

Using Tricylics for a Peaceful Death

The drugs have several characteristics that make them useful as reliable and lethal drugs. In particular they exhibit cardiotoxic and central nervous system (CNS) effects. CNS symptoms include sedation and coma, but it is the cardiotoxic effects that reduce cardiac output, lower blood pressure and disrupt cardiac rhythm that bring about death.

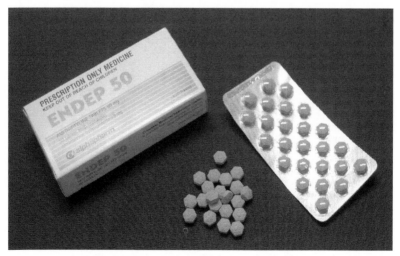

Fig 12.1 The tricyclic antidepressant amitriptyline

The toxic effects are accentuated if the drug is rapidly absorbed from the gut and this occurs in the alkaline environment of the small intestine. Preparation as a drink facilitates this, as does the use of an anti-emetic like metoclopramide (Maxolon - see Chapter 9) which speeds gastric emptying.

Amitriptyline is one of the most sedating of the TCAs and particularly useful as a lethal drug. The drug is marketed as Endep or Elavil tablets. The amount required is 5gm.

Preparation of Amitriptyline

The drug is usually packaged as tablets in 10, 25, 50 or 100mg amounts (Fig 12.1) and is usually supplied in packets of 50 tablets. Two packets of 50mg tablets is (100 x 50mg) or 5gm of the drug.

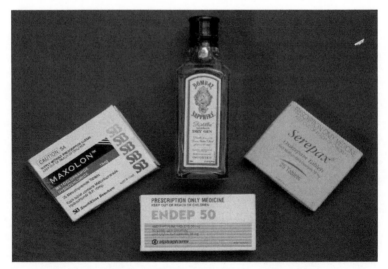

Fig 12.2 Amitriptyline with metocloptamide, oxazepam and Gin

For a peaceful death, open the blister packs and place 100 of the 50mg tablets in a glass. Add enough water to cover the drug and with gentlyagitation allow the drug to dissolve.

Take 6 x 10mg metoclopramide tablets and wait 40 minutes before drinking the dissolved amitriptyline. Follow this with 10 or more benzodiazepine sleeping tablets, then finish by taking alcohol to potentiate the action of the drug, and take away the bitter drug after-taste.

Note: Although amitriptyline is a strong sedative and sleep will quickly result, it is common to include a benzodiazepine sleeping drug after taking the amitriptyline and before the whisky. Serapax (oxazepam) is useful (see Chapter 11).

Once the drink has been consumed, settle back and take the alcohol. The drug cocktail will work quickly inducing sleep in about 15 minutes. Sleep will then deepen as consciousness is lost and the cardiotoxic properties of the drug bring about death. This period can vary and it is a good idea to have prepared a situation where there is no likelihood of disturbance for a period of up to 24 hours. (Fig12.2 & Video).

How does Amitriptyline score on the RP test?

Exit has no confirmed reports of failure using this regime and it rates 9/10 for Reliability. The time before sleep occurs is longer than with the barbiturates and this can cause anxiety. Peacefulness (7/10).

In the minor categories: Availability 2/5. It can be a difficult drug to acquire. Preparation is more complicated than with other ingestibles (Pr=3/5). The drug is undetectable - unless there is an autopsy. There is nothing about the death that suggests the use of this drug - the person looks as though they have died of a cardiac arrest (which they have - D=3/5). The process is however slow (Sp=2/5) and the drug has a moderate shelf life (St=3/5). The drug presents no risk to others (Sa=5/5). Total 34 or 68%

RP Test for Amitriptyline

Criteria	Score
Reliability	*9/10*
Peacefulness	*7/10*
Availability	*2/5*
Preparation	*3/5*
Undetectability	*3/5*
Speed	*2/5*
Safety	*5/5*
Storage	*3/5*
Total	*34 (68%)*

Insulin

There has been a lot of recent interest in the use of Insulin to provide a peaceful death. Reasons for this are easy to understand. In developed nations there is a huge growth in the numbers of people with Type 2 diabetes, and a corresponding increase in the number of people with ready access to this drug. An additional factor is the common chronic complications that often accompany severe forms of this disease. These symptoms can often so limit a person's quality of life, that the option of a peaceful death is sought.This drives interest in the use of this drug.

What is Insulin, and how can it end life

Insulin is produced in the pancreas and controls sugar levels in the body. If the pancreas fails (type 1 diabetes), or if the insulin produced fails to have the expected effect (type 2 diabetes), blood sugar levels (BSL) rise and disease results. Synthetic insulin can then be used to drive down the BSL to normal levels. However, if an overdose of this drug is taken, the blood sugar can be pushed dangerously low, and diabetic hypoglycemic coma and death result.

A hypoglycemic death from Insulin overdose, where the brain is starved from sugar, can be relatively peaceful. Initial symptoms of confusion and incoordination (often confused with drunkenness) can lead on to a rapid loss of consciousness.

Significant problems using Insulin

The biggest problem with using the drug in this way is that Insulin must be injected. As yet there are no oral forms of the drug.

The problems of intravenous administration have been described in Chapter 9, and although insulin can also (and usually is) given by subcutaneous injection, trying to administer an excess of 1000U of the rapid acting form of this drug, by the subcutaneous method can be practically impossible.

The other issue is that the growing number of people with access to this drug have the form of the disease where their bodies are unresponsive to the drug (Type 2 diabetes). While 1000U administered rapidly might peacefully end the life of a non-diabetic, those with the disease need to be much more careful.

In theory, one can pre-sensitise oneself, by taking alcohol (which restricts the body's emergency release of sugar), fasting, and by the administration of a significant dose of oral hypoglycemics before the insulin is injected. (eg ~50mg Glimepiride), the risks and uncertainties of the administration of a large subcutaneous injection remain.

In Summary

Not reliable enough to recommend if subcutaneous injection is the only method of administration available.

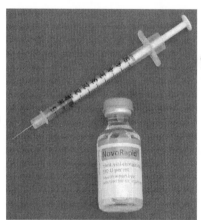

Fig 12.3 'NovoRapid' rapid acting insulin ampoule, 1000U in 10ml with 0.5ml syringe for subcutaneous administration

NOTE: 20 full syringes would need to be quickly injected to administer 1000U

13

Drug Options - Nembutal

I am hoping to get access to your 'peaceful pill' – not for immediate use, but to have on hand should my health deteriorate too much in the future. Arthur, 77 years

Introduction

The barbiturate Sodium Pentobarbital is the drug that comes closest to the concept of the Peaceful Pill. Exit defines the 'Peaceful Pill' as a pill, tablet or mixture that can be taken orally and that is guaranteed to provide a peaceful, dignified death at a time of one's choosing.

A Short History of Barbiturates

Sodium Pentobarbital or Nembutal as it is commonly called is an important and historically significant drug. Although Nembutal is one of over 50 barbiturate derivatives to have been used medically, it is the drug of choice when it comes to dignified, peaceful dying.

All Barbiturates are derivatives of barbituric acid which was first synthesized by Adolph von Bayer in 1864. A 'condensation' of malonic acid and urea, barbituric acid is said to have acquired its name after St Barbara's Day (4 December) - the day on which it is believed to have been discovered.

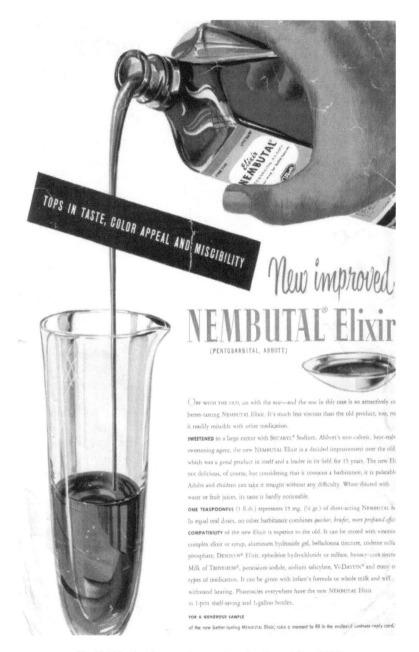

Fig 13.1 Nembutal women's magazine advertisment from 1950's

Other historians have speculated that the discovery may have been named after the chemist's favourite barmaid, Barbara. Either way, the name stuck and barbituric acid has enjoyed an infamous history ever since (Mendelson, 1980). Barbituric acid was found to have no physiological effect and it took another 40 years before chemists, Emil Fischer and Joseph von Mering, discovered that the introduction of two additional side-arms onto the molecule produced a range of compounds with marked physiological activity. It was only then that it became known that the nature of the sedative, hypnotic, or anaesthetic properties of the substance were determined by the characteristics of the side-arms attached.

The first of these di-substituted barbiturates was Veronal. Here two ethyl side-arms were added to produce diethyl-barbituric acid a weak hypnotic/ depressant which was marketed by the Bayer company as 'Veronal' in 1904. This was followed by phenobarbital (Luminal) in 1913. While barbituric acid is a German discovery, during the First World War when German shipping was blockaded, American chemists made use of the 'Trading with the Enemy Act,' to copy the work of the Germans and manufacture their own modifications of barbituric acid.

Barbiturate Sleeping Pills

In the first half of the 20th Century, barbiturates were manufactured around the world, with production peaking in the 1950s. By then there were more than 20 marketed forms of barbiturates, with most sold as sleeping tablets.

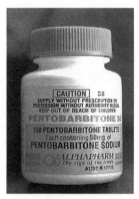

Fig 13.2: Pentobarbital (Nembutal) sleeping tablets

Along with the original Veronal, there was Barbital, Amytal, Seconal, Soneryl, Nembutal and several others.

While these barbiturates were highly effective sleeping tablets, a significant problem was the very serious side-effect associated with their overdose - death. This was found to be especially true if the pills were taken with alcohol. Many famous people have died - some deliberately, some inadvertently - from an overdose of barbiturates. Marilyn Monroe, Judy Garland and Jimmy Hendrix are a few.

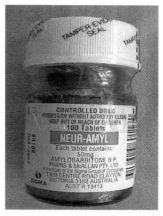

Fig 13.3: Amylobarbital (Amytal) sleeping tablets

Barbiturates as Drugs of Abuse

In the 1960s, the image of barbiturates suffered further when they were found to be useful mood-altering drugs. At this time, the depressant effect of the drugs was exploited. By carefully adjusting the dose, a desirable soporific and tranquil state could be achieved and they became known as 'downers.' As downers, barbiturates would often be intermixed with 'uppers' - drugs like amphetamines. This type of usage led to a set of slang street terms for these drugs such as 'Pink Ladies', 'Yellow Bullets', 'Peanuts' and 'Dolls' (from Barbie dolls) (Mendelson, 1980).

With only a small margin of safety in dose between the desired sleep, euphoria and death, there was considerable danger associated with the prescription of these drugs. History shows they fell out of favour with the medical profession once newer, safer sleeping tablets became available.

The Advent of Non-barbiturate Sleeping Pills

The first of the new class of sleeping drugs (the benzodiazepines) was diazepam (Valium), which became available in the early 1960s. These drugs were welcomed by the medical profession as a safe alternative to the barbiturate sleeping tablets. At this time there were many prescribed forms of barbiturates on the market but with the introduction of these new benzodiazepines, the use of the barbiturates steadily declined.

By the mid 1990s in countries like Australia, there were just two barbiturate sleeping tablets left, amylobarbital (Amytal) and pentobarbital (Nembutal). Nembutal was withdrawn with little notice in 1998 with Amytal following suit in 2003. Today, the only barbiturate commonly prescribed by doctors is the slow-acting Phenobarbital. This drug still finds a niche in medicine as an anti-convulsant, but is a poor substitute to the specific barbiturate sleeping tablets in providing a reliable, peaceful death.

Barbiturate Use in Veterinary Practice

The veterinary use of the barbiturates has persisted. Nembutal, in particular, is used as an agent for euthanasia. A large dose delivered intravenously, quickly and peacefully ends an animal's life. This green-dyed form of the drug, known as Lethabarb or Valabarb, is also known as 'the green dream.'

A sterile form of Nembutal has also persisted as a useful complete anaesthetic agent that can quickly render an animal unconscious for surgery. Pentobarbital continues to play a role in veterinary practice to this day even though its use by the medical profession has all but disappeared. A development that has led to a resurrection of these outdated drugs is their increasing use as the drugs of choice for voluntary euthanasia (and state-sanctioned executions in some states of the US).

Nembutal in Countries where Assisted Dying is Legal

Nembutal is the drug of choice in countries where VE and Assisted Suicide are legal and is used in The Netherlands, Belgium, Switzerland and the US states of Oregon, Washington, Montana and Vermont.

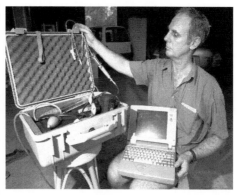

When the *Rights of the Terminally Ill Act* was passed in the Northern Territory, I had the challenge of deciding which drug or substance would produce the most humane, peaceful reliable death.

Fig 13.4: The 'Deliverance' euthanasia machine

After much research and consultation - a process that even saw us seeking information about the drugs used for execution in the US - a decision was made to sanction the use of a large intravenous or oral dose of Nembutal.

The four people who died using the *ROTI Act* all injected themselves with Nembutal (with the help of the Deliverance Machine, now on display in the British Science Museum).
http://en.wikipedia.org/wiki/File:Euthanasia_machine_(Australia).JPG)

While these people could also have simply drunk the liquid Nembutal, each preferred intravenous administration. When delivered in this way, loss of consciousness is almost immediate (seconds), with death following a short time later.

Drinking Nembutal is often the preferred option and means no other person need be involved in administration. For example, in the state of Oregon in the US, a doctor is only allowed to *prescribe* as opposed to *administer* a 10 gm oral dose of barbiturates to a patient. The patient must drink the drug themselves. In Switzerland, too, it is the client who must administer the drug him/her self. In Holland and Belgium, it is lawful to provide barbiturates as an injection to a dying patient. The drug used in each these places is Nembutal.

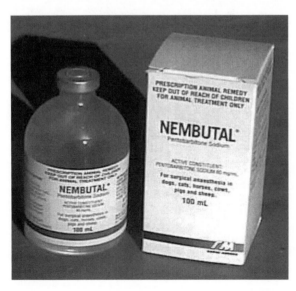

Fig 13.5:
Sterile veterinary
Nembutal

How Barbiturates Work

Barbiturates effect the action of the brain chemical GABA in that they enhance the effect of GABA on the brain, and may even act in its place. GABA slows the activity of the brain. Enhancing its action causes sedation and sleep. In larger doses, the barbiturate may even replace the GABA in the brain. An overdose of a barbiturate can depress brain function so severely that respiration ceases and the person dies.

As discussed above, the depressant effect of barbiturates can be useful in counteracting the irritability and paranoia that can result from the use of amphetamines. Barbiturates have also been reported to be effective in alleviating the symptoms of heroin withdrawal. In the 1960s, injecting drug users were reported to have substituted barbiturates for opiates like heroin and methadone if such drugs were not available.

Available Forms of Nembutal

For human use, Nembutal was extensively marketed as sleeping tablets or capsules in the 1950s & 1960s. Even though Nembutal disappeared off the market over a decade ago, many people have old stocks which are still potent. One hundred of these capsules (100 x 100mg = 10gm of barbiturate) is a lethal dose.

Barbiturates are also well absorbed rectally and some countries have marketed forms of suppositories. 'Nova Rectal' in Canada is one such example. Sterile ampoules of injectable Nembutal for intramuscular and intravenous administration as a hypnotic, anti-convulsant and pre-operative sedative still find a small place in medicine in some countries including the US.

The veterinary forms of the drug are also still used in either the sterile injectable form for anaesthesia, or a non-sterile form (Valabarb or Lethabarb) for animal euthanasia.

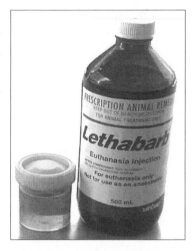

The sterile form of this veterinary barbiturate (fig 13.5) is marketed in small, sealed 100ml bottles that are protected with a metal seal. This metal cap makes tampering obvious. The Nembutal inside is a clear liquid with concentration of 60 mg/ml. Each 100ml bottle

Fig 13.6: Non-sterile coloured veterinary Nembutal (Lethabarb)

has a total of 6 gm of Nembutal - enough to provide a peaceful death.

Non-sterile Nembutal liquid ('Lethabarb', Fig 13.6) is used for animal euthanasia, is colour dyed for safety, and has a much higher concentration of barbiturate (300mg/ml). 30ml taken orally is lethal.

Since 2010, the powdered form of the drug (sodium pentobarbital) has become available as an assay-grade laboratory reagent. For details of this useful form of the drug - see Chapter 14.

Pentobarb & Phenobarb – Confusing Names

Nembutal is the commercial or trade name for the barbiturate whose chemical name is pentobarbital ('pent-o-barb-it-al'). This drug is different to another barbiturate called phenobarbital. Phenobarbital is a slow-acting drug, used predominantly as an anti-convulsant to stabilise people suffering from epilepsy.

While phenobarb can be lethal in overdose, it has a much slower action than Nembutal and is not an ideal method for self-deliverance. These two barbiturates should not be confused.

Sources of Nembutal

In most western countries there are now no medically prescribed barbiturate sleeping tablets. What remains in the public consciousness, however, is the belief that an overdose of sleeping tablets - any sleeping tablet – will cause death. This misconception leads to many failed suicide attempts as elderly or seriously ill people often stockpile, then take, large numbers of modern, non-lethal sleeping tablets.

Let us be clear. There is *no point* in asking your doctor for sleeping tablets if you plan to end your life. Tablets obtained this way *will not* be barbiturates and the drugs obtained will be unlikely, even in significant overdose, to cause death.

The commonest source of life-ending barbiturates in most western countries is the veterinary profession, and even this supply is likely to diminish in time. There is no legitimate or plausible reason for a vet to provide this drug to any member of the public. You can hardly tell your vet that you're planning to operate on the cat this weekend!

Nembutal and Vets

Veterinary Nembutal has been used by vets to euthanase animals or as an anaesthetic in surgery for many decades. Before 1998, when Nembutal was still being prescribed by doctors, it may just have been possible to argue that your insomnia was so bad that only the rare and dangerous Nembutal could help you get

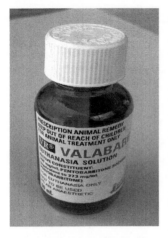

Fig 13.7: Non-sterile veterinary Nembutal (Valabarb)

a good night's sleep. But there is simply no excuse one can give a vet to obtain this drug!

If a vet were ever to provide Nembutal - knowing what the person has in mind - they could face a charge of assisting a suicide. De-registration and a prison term would be the likely consequence. In 2001 the Australian Veterinary Board became concerned about the increasing use of veterinary Nembutal as a human euthanasia option and put out a warning to its members urging caution in the storage and use of the drug. (see *Veterinary Surgeons Board, 2003*).

Exit knows of only a handful of cases where seriously ill people have been able to obtain Nembutal from their Vet. When there is public mention of this possibility, the Veterinary Associations have reacted quickly denying the practice.

Moves to further restrict the use of veterinary Nembutal has meant that the anaesthetic form of the drug (see Fig 13.5) is becoming more difficult to obtain. This is the form of the drug favoured by those wanting it for their own use, comforted by the fact that it comes in a clearly-labelled sterile sealed bottles.

The non-sterile green dyed form is more concentrated than its clear counterpart. Marketed as Valabarb (Fig 13.7) or Lethabarb (Fig 13.6) the concentration of this type of pentobarbital is 300mg/ml (five times higher than in the sterile anaesthetic form). A single 30ml sample will contain 10gm of Nembutal and be lethal. This non-sterile green liquid needs to be decanted from a larger 500ml bottle. If drunk it can stain the lips and tongue.

With such staining it is unlikely that an attending doctor will cite natural causes on the death certificate.

A Case Study in Nembutal

When asked about Nembutal at Exit workshops, I tell people that it can be very handy to know a vet. Some time ago, I was making a clinic visit to the bedside of Harry, a dying patient. With his wife at his side Harry asked me about 'the best drugs', the ones that would let him peacefully end his own life.

I explained that the 'best' drug was Nembutal, but that this was only available from a vet. 'How many vets do you know really well' I asked, 'ones that will risk jail helping you?' His silence answered my question, and we went on to talk about other more easily available, but less effective, drugs.

After the visit, I left the bedroom and had a cup of tea in the kitchen with Harry's wife, Esme. Tentatively she said, 'you know when you asked about knowing a vet?' I looked at her, confused. She went on 'well, I knew a vet, very well indeed.' I waited, not knowing what was to follow. She continued. 'In fact, some time back I had an affair with a vet. My husband knows nothing about it, and I want to keep it that way. But that vet owes me some bloody big favours and I'm going to call them in!'

A few weeks later, Harry died of his disease. I heard that Esme did indeed call in the favour, obtaining the 100ml bottle of liquid Nembutal. She told me that the bottle sat in the bedroom with Harry during his last weeks and that he drew immense comfort from knowing it was there. As he faced every new day, he was reassured by the knowledge that if the day became too difficult, he could leave at any time. Indeed, the presence of the drug prolonged Harry's life.

The number of people who have a vet as their best friend, a friend prepared to risk jail for them is very small. There has only been a handful of occasions when I have seen help provided in this way, and Harry's was one of them. Perhaps the question put to patients should be rephrased, perhaps I should be asking 'have you ever had an affair with a vet?' When I told this story at a recent public meeting, one elderly woman shouted back 'I wish you'd told me that 40 years ago.'

Nembutal and the Black Market

Exit receives occasional reports of people paying a very high price on the black market for Nembutal. Desperate for the drug, some have paid over $5000 for a single 100ml bottle of veterinary Nembutal. This same bottle would retail to a vet for less than $50. Despite the huge potential profit to a dealer, Nembutal is rarely found this way. The usual laws of supply and demand that govern the illegal drug trade do not apply, as no one will ever want more than one bottle of this drug. Supply chains do not therefore develop.

The Nembutal that does find its way on to the street is usually in the form of the sterile veterinary liquid. It is presumed that it is obtained when veterinary clinics are broken into by people looking for tradeable veterinary steroids.

If the seal and labelling of a Nembutal bottle is intact and the expiry date not exceeded, the drug is likely to be effective. Nevertheless, one is advised to test the substance if planning to use such sources. The Exit barbiturate test kit is available at: *http://bit.ly/9swOxk*

The Exit Test Kit enables people who have acquired liquid Nembutal to self-test the drug.

Note: The 'Exit Spot Test Kit' provides qualitative evidence of the presence of the drug. The Exit Dilution Purity Test Kit (launched in 2013) provides a quantitative test process (ie. drug concentration and strength) as a home test.

The Shelf Life of Liquid Nembutal

Event though most liquid Nembutal will have an expiry date of around two years, this is one substance that is known to remain effective for much longer. If stored in a cool place and kept in its sterile, sealed bottle, liquid Nembutal can be expected to have a shelf-life of many years.

A detailed discussion of the shelf life of both liquid and powdered Nembutal can be found in Chapter 15.

Nembutal - Summary

The barbiturate pentobarbital (Nembutal) is the best euthanasia drug and comes closest to the concept of the Peaceful Pill. In countries where it is lawful to help someone to die and any drug or substance could be used, the choice is always Nembutal.

Yet Nembutal is a hard drug to obtain with doctors in most western countries no longer able/ willing to prescribe the drug. Nembutal's restricted use by vets makes it increasingly difficult to access.

However, Nembutal can be obtained from overseas, in South America, SE Asia, and in powdered form from China. The next chapter gives a detailed outline of where to go and how to buy Nembutal. This information changes frequently and is regularly updated for the online version of *The Peaceful Pill eHandbook.*

Exit RP Test - Nembutal

Criteria	Score
Reliability	*10/10*
Peacefulness	*10/10*
Availability	*2/5*
Preparation	*5/5*
Undetectability	*4/5*
Speed	*4/5*
Safety	*5/5*
Storage	*4/5*
Total Score	*44 (88%)*

14

Obtaining Nembutal

Introduction

For many years now, Nembutal has been available in a number of countries. In most western countries, however, the drug remains heavily restricted with anyone importing drug almost inevitably *breaking the law*. Where and how one can obtain Nembutal is a moveable feast. In recent years, solid sources of supply have emerged in countries as diverse as Peru and China. This information continues to change constantly.

In this chapter the following issues are covered:

- Types of Nembutal for sale
- Drug Labelling
- Legal Issues
- Nembutal over the Internet: Mexico
- Nembutal over the Internet: China
- Tested Chinese Suppliers
- Current Chinese Suppliers
- The TOR Router, Bitcoins & The Silk Road
- Nembutal over the counter: Mexico, Peru, Bolivia, SE Asia

Since this *Handbook* was first published in 2006, Exit has established a global network of travellers who have purchased Nembutal around the world. This allows value feedback to be collated and later published. Exit acknowledges that the availability of Nembutal *can and does change without warning.* Old stores close and new stores open. Websites appear and disappear, seemingly overnight. As the well-known expats Carol Schmidt, Norma Hair and Rolly Brook write of Mexico:

> *what is true today may not be true tomorrow, or true to the border agent in the next lane, or even to the same agent before and after lunch ... the authors can provide no guarantees that what we publish today won't change tomorrow ...*

As one US tourist to Mexico put it:

> *Mexican border towns are depressed and scruffy-looking and it is almost always possible to get just about anything you want. This is all the more so given the currently depressed economy -- and this is important to remember. No matter what the government may do, it will always be possible to get Nembutal here unless its manufacture gets prohibited. How to get it is the challenge!*

In past years, most people visited countries such as Mexico, Peru or Thailand to purchase Nembutal over-the-counter. In recent years, the Internet has largely taken over. While Nembutal continues to be available in such countries, the Internet has emerged to offer altogether new options for obtaining Nembutal which remains best drug for a reliable and peaceful death at a time of one's choosing.

Types of Nembutal on Sale

Nembutal (Pentobarbital Sodium) can be purchased both over-the-counter and by mail order, either in solution as a veterinary liquid, or as the white crystalline salt. Rarely the drug can still be found as tablets or capsules for human use as a sleeping agent.

The liquid form is a veterinary product that is used for animal anaesthesia and usually packaged as a sterile liquid in either 50ml or 100ml bottles. It is always at the same concentration of 60mg/ml (ie a 50ml/100ml bottle contains 3gm/6gm of Nembutal).

The white crystalline solid powder is the form that is generally available from China.

Nembutal tablets for human use are still available in some countries (eg. Thailand) on prescription as a sleeping tablets.

Drug Labelling

Where veterinary Nembutal is sold over-the-counter in liquid form, it is marketed under a range of retail names. The key ingredient to look for on the label is 'Pentobarbital Sodium'.

In Mexico, veterinary Nembutal is sold over-the-counter and online and labelled as: *Anestesal, Pisabental, Barbithal, Sedalforma, Sedalforte, Pentovet, Pentomax* (see Fig 14.1 - 14.9). In Peru and Bolivia, veterinary Nembutal is retailed as *Halatal* or *Penta-Hypnol* (see Fig 14.28 - 14.30)   In Thailand it is marketed as *Nembutal.*(see Fig 14.31)

Mail order Chinese Nembutal is sold as reagent grade 'Sodium Pentobarbital', CAS No. 57-33-0 (see Fig 14.14 - 14.17).

Legal Considerations

If you choose to purchase Nembutal in another country, you should be aware that importation of the drug back to your country of origin is likely to be *against the law*. If you take this course of action you will be breaking the law.

The legal penalties for the importation of Nembutal vary depending on the country. In some jurisdictions, the importation of a single bottle of Nembutal will be dealt with summarily (by a single Magistrate or Judge). In others it may be referred to the criminal courts, with the case heard by a judge and jury.

In general, the way in which the importation of a border-controlled substance such as Nembutal is dealt with by authorities will depend on the amount and purity of the substance that you are alleged to have imported. The offence of importing a border-controlled drug will depend on how authorities measure the amount imported, and whether it can be classified as 'marketable', 'trafficable' or 'commercial' in quantity? Classifications will vary depending on jurisdiction, with legal penalties varying accordingly.

The seriousness/ criminality of an alleged importation of Nembutal will also depend on the drug's purity. In some countries, the 'marketable quantity' of Nembutal (ie. the amount which makes the importation of this drug a serious offence) might be 50gm. While one bottle of veterinary Nembutal contains only 6gm of pentobarbital sodium (with the remaining mixture being alcohol), the authorities may have the power to charge the person with importing a full 100gm/ 100ml contained even in the bottle, even though only 6% of the mixture is the actual border-controlled drug.

Thus, any person who chooses to import a single bottle of Nembutal may find themselves facing severe penalties if

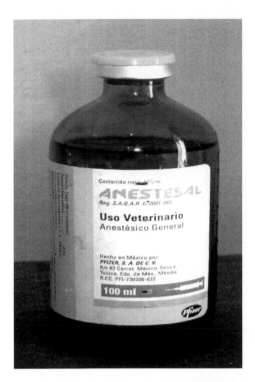

Fig 14.1: Mexican veterinary sterile Nembutal: Anestesal

Fig 14.2: Mexican veterinary sterile Nembutal: Sedal-Vet

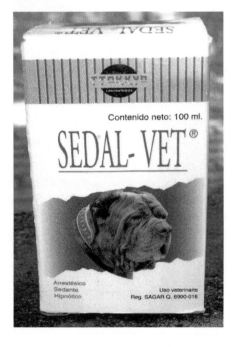

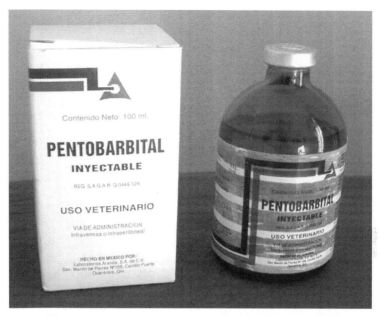

Fif 14.3: Mexican veterinary sterile Nembutal: Pentobarbital Injectible

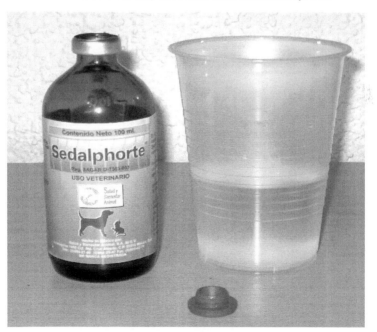

Fig 14.4: Mexican veterinary sterile Nembutal: Sedalphorte

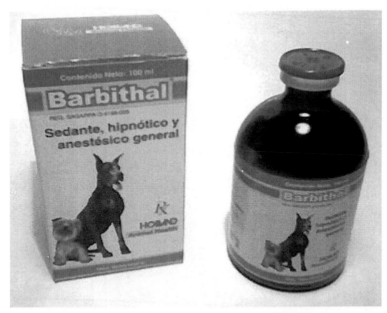

Fig 14.5: Mexican veterinary sterile Nembutal: Barbithal

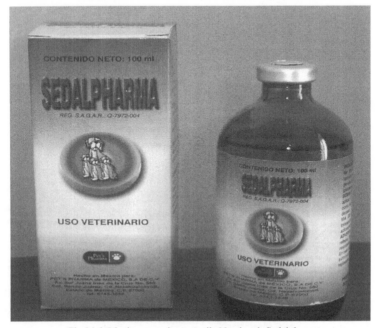

Fig 14.6: Mexican veterinary sterile Nembutal: Sedalpharma

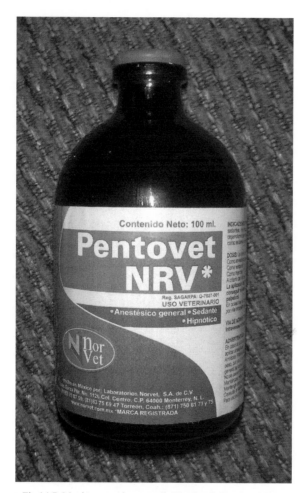

Fig 14.7: Mexican veterinary sterile Nembutal: Pentovet NRV

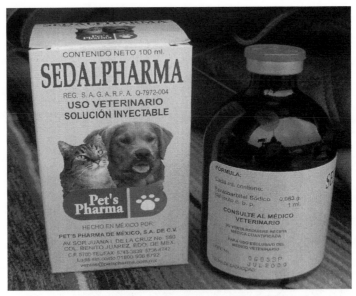

Fig 14.8: Mexican veterinary sterile Nembutal: Sedalpharma

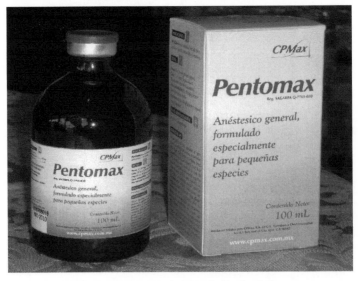

Fig 14.9: Mexican veterinary sterile Nembutal: Pentomax

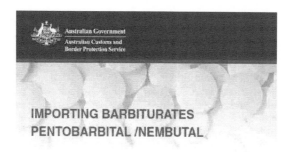

**IMPORTING BARBITURATES
PENTOBARBITAL /NEMBUTAL**

WHAT IS IT?

Pentobarbital is a short acting barbiturate which is commonly sold under several names including Nembutal and Sedalphone. Phenobarbital has been used both in animals and humans as a sedative, hypnotic, anticonvulsant and anaesthetic drug. These drugs are available in both liquid and tablet form.

Recent media reports have stated that people have sought to illegally import Nembutal to assist in suicide. Some euthanasia groups have also advocated purchasing the drug overseas and encouraged travellers to conceal it from Customs and Border Protection on their return home. Be aware that importing barbiturates without permission is a serious offence and offenders will be referred to the Australian Federal Police.

WHAT ARE THE RESTRICTIONS?

Barbiturates are listed as a prohibited import under Item 18, Schedule 4 (Regulation 5) of the *Customs (Prohibited Imports) Regulations 1956*. Barbiturates are a group of medicines with many legitimate applications and there is a permission regime in place to allow for legitimate importations. Commercial importers need to be licensed and have written permission to import into Australia. Permits are issued to commercial importers through the Office of Chemical Safety and Environmental Health (OCSEH), within the Department of Health and Ageing.

Incoming passengers into Australia on a ship or aircraft carrying barbiturates for the purpose of treating a medical condition or treating a passenger who is in their care are able to carry a three month supply of medication, provided that the passenger has a prescription or a letter from their medical practitioner. Australian residents must carry a prescription from an Australian registered medical practitioner.

WHY ARE THESE RESTRICTIONS IN PLACE?

Barbiturates are classed as a Prescription Only Medication under the Standard for the Uniform Scheduling of Medicines and Poisons (SUSMP) and can only be used or supplied on the order of persons permitted by State or Territory legislation (medical practitioner) to prescribe and should be made available to patients on prescription only. **Use of Pentobarbital without medical supervision can potentially be dangerous to health, toxic or poisonous.**

HOW IS PERMISSION SOUGHT?

Licenses and permits are not granted to individuals for the purpose of obtaining medications for personal use, or to assist with suicide. If you are an individual wanting to access medications that are prohibited on import, you should consult your doctor. If you have a legitimate need for Pentobarbital, your doctor may be able to apply through the Special Access Scheme (SAS) administered by the Therapeutic Goods Administration (TGA). Once approval is granted by the TGA, the applicant (medical practitioner) will require a permit from OCSEH for clearance on importation.

PENALTIES

Barbiturates are listed as a border controlled drug under the *Criminal Code 1995* and their illegal importation may attract criminal sanctions. Penalties range from imprisonment and/or fines up to $825,000.

Fig 14.10 Australian Government publication March 2011

the amount is deemed to be 'marketable.' One way a minor importation offence can turn into a significant crime would be to tell authorities the drug is for another person, rather than for personal use, as this is admitting of drug trafficking.

Note: Drugs such as barbiturates are often of secondary concern to authorities who seem far more interested in substances such as cocaine, cannabis, amphetamines and party drugs such as ecstasy and GHB. It is the distribution of these latter drugs, rather than barbiturates which is linked with international organised crime syndicates. The barbiturates have lost their appeal as drugs of addiction/ abuse and feature little in blackmarket trade. After all, one person will only ever need 10gm of Nembutal.

Despite this, the efficacy of Exit International in promoting the acquisition of this drug by the elderly and sick has led the Australian government to issue a statement in March 2011 that refers to 'some euthanasia groups ... advocat[ing] purchasing the drug overseas and encouraging travellers to conceal it from Customs and Border Protection on their return home'. The document seems designed to discourage people from taking this course and refers to the penalties for importing a border-controlled drug as ranging from imprisonment to fines up to A$850,000. (Fig 12.10)

http://www.customs.gov.au/webdata/resources/files/ImportingBarbiturates. PDF

Exit has put considerable effort into ensuring that readers of *The Handbook* and *Peaceful Pill Handbook* have all information necessary to make informed choices. We make it clear that in providing this information we are not encouraging the reader to break the law.

Legal Issues (Cont) - Case Study

To date, Exit knows of only one person who has been charged with importation offences anywhere in the world. This person was a member of Exit (Ann) from Melbourne, Australia. Ann was charged with importation of two bottles of Nembutal after her consignment was intercepted by Customs and referred to the Australian Federal Police (AFP) in early 2009.

The first Ann was aware that her Nembutal would not be arriving was when the AFP came to her home, and served a search warrant. At her court hearing in April a year later, she pleaded guilty. Since this was her first offence, the Magistrate issued her with a fine of $500, a 12 month good behaviour bond and ordered she pay $1000 to the court fund. No conviction was recorded.
See: http://bit.ly/bECnzG

Note: In the US, this product is listed in the Federal Controlled Substances Act under DEA schedule II.

Nembutal Over the Internet: USA

In recent times, new websites claiming to sell 'pharmeceutical grade', sterile liquid Nembutal - manufactured by Oak Pharmeceuticals - are merging on the Internet.

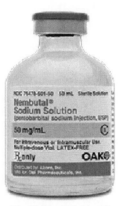

One of these websites is called 'Buy Nembutal' and can be found at:*http:// buynembutal.webs.com/* Beware! Those who have dealt with this site say it is a scam.

In June 2013, Steve from California said:

Fig 14.11a: Oak Liquid Nembutal 50ml bottle

I think this link is intended to fleece people who are faced with a difficult life decision. I was given a price quote for powdered Nembutal by a Garry Laudrup and instructed to send the funds by MoneyGram to a Virginia address.

The next day Garry said they had an insufficient quantity of Nembutal and that I should change the MoneyGram to an Ivanova in Macedonia and that the Nembutal would be shipped from there. After inquiries about shipment details, I was informed that the shipment would be by EMS and demanding a "refundable" insurance payment of an additional $500.

I have sent an email to Garry Laudrup demanding an explanation for this apparent fraud. I assumed that my initial payment was at risk, but the scale of the fraud seems to have no bounds.

Nembutal Over the Internet: Mexico

For several years, Exit has been aware of a mail-order Mexican
Nembutal at the Metroflog site of:
http://www.metroflog.com/tyler_durden_nemb

Over the years, Exit has received on-going feedback on this
website.   A selection is included.

Fig 14.11a:
Mexican internet
Nembutal website

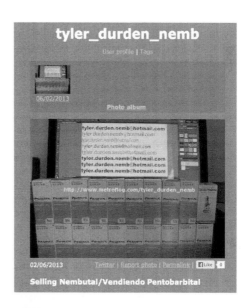

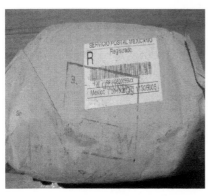

Fig 14.11b:
Liquid Nembutal
as shipped from
Mexico

September 2013
I received my packages as promised. He is very reliable. He tells you what he is going to do and then does it. I am very grateful to him for this service.
Sam, Oregon

June 2013
Hello, I just want to inform you that I used information from *The Peaceful Pill Handbook* and received excellent service. He responded quickly and the package came in good condition after only 10 days after shipping. He responded promptly to emails, gave good directions, and had a sensitive tone and manner.
 I am very appreciative of Exit's publications.
Sylvia, Florida

April 2013
My email exchange and subsequent transaction with this contact was a smooth, straight forward and professional process. The package took just under two weeks after payment was made. The bottle arrived padded within its small envelope and in one piece.
Chris, NY

March 2013
I am from Turkey. I bought 1 bottle of 100 cc/ml Nembutal. He is a very helpful, trustworth and kind man. For one bottle I paid US$450. The package arrived on 22 March, 4 weeks after shipment. By the way thanks to the Peaceful Pill Handbook.
Henry, Turkey

A new development in the shipping of Nembutal from Mexico is the inclusion of anti-emetic drugs. In many countries, these are only available on prescription although in Mexico metoclopramide is available over-the-counter for around $3 a pack. As Lois commented, 'it is a really nice touch'.

Nembutal Over the Internet: China

In recent years, powder Nembutal has been widely available by mail order from China. *The New York Times* has reported that this has been possible because chemical companies are relatively unregulated by the Chinese authorities. In comparison, drug companies are highly regulated, due largely to the multi-million dollar industry of drug counterfeit industry that the Chinese Government is attempting to stamp out.
http://topics.nytimes.com/top/news/international/series/toxicpipeline/index. html

Marketed as reagent grade pentobarbital sodium (CAS No. 57-33-0) this water-soluble, white crystalline solid is stated as having a purity of better than 99%. Administration is a matter of dissolving ~10gm of the powder in ~ 50ml of water and drinking.

While the source companies have long claimed that their product is pure, it was not until mid 2011 that Exit was able to verify a number of samples, through laboratory testing. If the powder is analysed to be pure, and if ingested in the recommended amounts, Chinese Nembutal powder will (not might) lead to a reliable and peaceful death. (See Chapter 15 for the full discussion of the laboratory test results undertaken by Exit).

The cost of Chinese powder Nembutal has fluctuated markedly since it was first available. Some folk have paid as little as US$260 for 20gms. Others have paid US$900 for the same amount. To date, payment has predominantly via Western Union and sometimes by Paypal. Delivery to the US and Australia has been within 3 days of orders being placed in some cases but generally 10 - 20 days.

The minimum lethal drug dose is 6gms. If the substance is pure, a purchase of 25gm of 95% pure sodium pentobarbital is more than enough for two adults.

In 2013, the product tends to be shipped flat-packed (see Figs 14.15 - 14.17).. In 2011 - 2012 the standard packaging was small plastic screw-top containers containing 12 gms in each (see Figs 14.12 & 14.13).

The Current Status of Chinese Nembutal

Over recent years, more than 14 different Chinese chemical companies have sold Nembutal. Exit's independent laboratory testing has consistently found the product to contain purities of greater than 95%. While no contaminated or adulterated samples have been found to date, this could change and is the reason Exit International has launched a mobile quantitative drug testing service (see Chapter 15 for details).

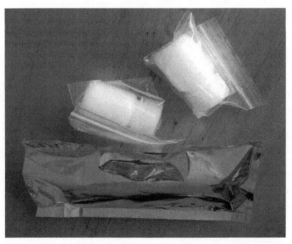

Fig 14.12: Powder Nembutal as shipped from China

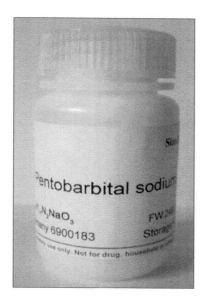

Fig 14.13: Nembutal from 3B
Scientific International

As with the availability of Nembutal in other countries, Chinese sources of Nembutal have been found to change rapidly, with previously reliable suppliers discontinuing and unknown others coming into the market. A summary of companies that have supplied or who claim to supply laboratory-grade sodium pentobarbital powder is listed below:

• Tested Suppliers (which may or may not still be shipping)
• Sellers (with a good track record of shipping/ delivery)

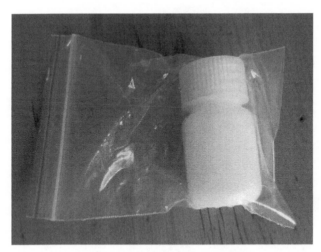

Fig 14.14: 12 gms powder from China

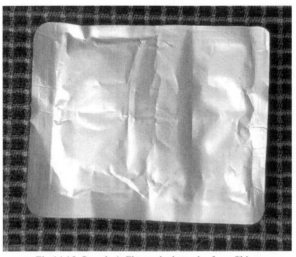

Fig 14.15: Sample 1: Flat-packed powder from China

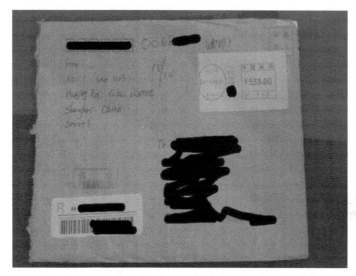

Fig 14.16: Sample 2: Envelope of flat-packed powder from China

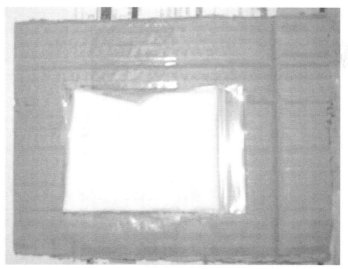

Fig 14.17: Sample 3: Package of flat-packed powder from China

Tested Chinese Suppliers (who may/may not be active)

Random samples from each of the suppliers listed below have undergone external, laboratory analysis. Results have shown 99% purity. However, whether these suppliers are continuing to ship Nembutal in 2013 remains unconfirmed.

Rundong Chemical, Quzhou
Email: *selley.dong@rundongchemical.com*

Haihang Industry Co
Email: *export001@haihangchem.com*

David Zhang
Email: *david.zhang57@gmail.com or david.zhang@hushmail.com*

Cherry Chemical, Hangzhou
Email: *cherrychemicals@gmail.com*

Nanjing Fubang Chemical Co. Ltd., Nanjing
Email: *Johnson0@fbchem.com or Johnson0@msn.cn*

Active Suppliers

Nanjing Fubang Chemical Co. Ltd., Nanjing
The contact at Nanjing is 'Johnson'.
The quoted price is US$250 for 25 gm, includes shipping.
Web: *www.fbchem.com*
Email: *Johnson0@fbchem.com or Johnson0@msn.cn*

Note: The importation of this drug in some countries can be a criminal offence. Exit recommends that folk check the laws of their local jurisdiction before proceeding down this path.

Nembutal on the Internet - Recent Trends

Since 2012, supplies of Chinese Nembutal have become less reliable. The sources listed as 'Tested' will ship to some on some days, but not to others. Persistence is often required, and occasionally one will lose their money.

There is also the increased enthusiasm on the part of Customs and Border Protection to restrict the importation of Nembutal. In Australia for example, the quantity of this drug seized has risen steeply over the past six months. *http://bit.ly/Zs8yLT*

While a number of Exit members have had their orders for Chinese Nembutal intercepted (and lost their money) we are unaware of any criminal charges being laid. One explanation for this is that the work required for a successful legal action exceeds any possible benefit. Prosecuting an elderly, hitherto law-abiding person for trying to import a one-off small quantity of the best euthanasia drug would attract considerable public interest and draw attention on to the failure of the political process in addressing end of life issues.

As is so often the case with sources of Nembutal, when one door shuts, another invariably opens. One strategy to emerge is the trend of travelling overseas to a country that has less interest in restricting the importation of this drug. Hong Kong and India are examples of this. Once there, an internet order can be made to a Chinese supplier, and delivery can be made at the vacation address,

Another strategy to recently emerge, and which does not require the expense and disruption of overseas travel, is to make use of the new security options that are now available on the Internet.

These strategies include:
- TOR 'onion routing' anonymizing software
- The use of Bitcoin Internet currency
- The Silk Road & other anonymous marketplaces

Using TOR client software ensures online anonymity.

TOR (onion routing) software is available free and 'is intended to protect users' personal privacy, freedom, and ability to conduct confidential business by keeping their internet activities from being monitored.' This is essential for those 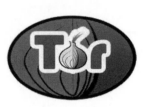 who desire a high level of privacy, removed from monitoring authorities, as they seek end of life drugs on the internet.

The necessary software can be downloaded free from:
https://www.torproject.org/

Using Bitcoin Virtual Currency for Payment

Bitcoin is a digital currency that uses free open source, peer-to-peer technology that 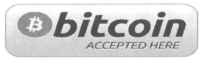 allows instant worldwide payments at a very low cost. This virtual currency enables pseudo-anonymous online payments. This is clearly useful when paying for items sourced anonymously using the TOR router.

To use Bitcoins, you will first need to choose an online 'wallet' to install on your computer or mobile phone. Upon installation, your wallet will generate a Bitcoin address, and allow you to purchase (and perhaps spend) your first Bitcoins in an anonymous way. Read more at *http://bitcoin.org/en/*

The 'Silk Road' Anonymous Marketplace

One important function of the TOR system is its ability to run location hidden services, websites that are not normally visible using regular browsers. One such hidden site is the on-line black 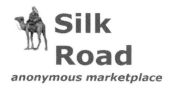 market 'Silk Road', best described as an anonymous market place. Access to The Silk Road is only available via TOR so this software must be installed and operating before one can explore the hidden site. Exit has been actively monitoring the Silk Road since its inception in 2011. At this stage (April 2013) Nembutal is not offered for purchase, but other barbiturates are available (Fig 14.17a). Exit expects to see Nembutal listed in the very near future.

For those contemplating using the TOR system, it is important to note that The Silk Road is only one of a number of hidden sites dealing in end of life drugs. Details of one particular service are currently being verified.

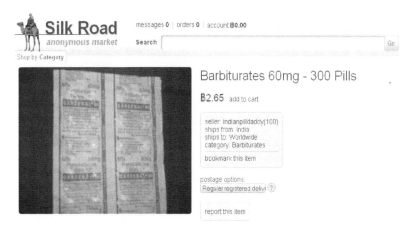

Fig 14.17a: Barbiturates from The Silk Road

Purchasing Nembutal in Person: Mexico

Over recent years, Exit staff and members have visited many Mexican cities with the purpose of researching sources of reliable end-of-life drugs. During this time, Exit has also received accounts from travellers regarding their experiences in this country. This section includes material that relates to travellers obtaining Nembutal in Mexico from 2010 to 2013 *only*.

Mazatlan

In 2011, Exit received its first report of the availability of Nembutal in the beachside resort of Mazatlan in the state of Sinaloa across from the Baja California peninsula. After unsuccessful attempts to purchase Nembutal in Tijuana the year before, an Exit member who we shall call 'Bob' took a vacation at Mazatlan.

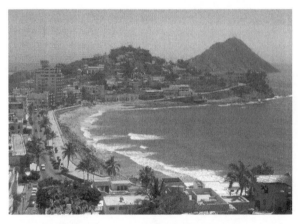

Fig 14.18: Playa Norte in Mazatlan, Mexico

His purchase was straight forward. The price was excellent at US$30 for a 100ml, sealed bottle with an expiry date of July 2013. The outlet where the purchase was made was the hole-in-the-wall El Arca de Noe (Noah's Ark) pharmacy located at:

Ejercito Mexicano No. 5
(near Playa Norte) area of Mazatlan

Bob says that he used the photos in the *Handbook* to explain to the sales attendant the precise drug he was after. The retail brand he purchased on this occasion was 'Sedalpharma'.

Playa del Carmen

In late 2010, Exit received its first report of the availability of Nembutal in the tourist resort town of Playa del Carmen. This Exit member wrote:

On my recent trip to Playa del Carmen we visited 5 or 6 shops and were always turned away; I was about to give up when the driver said he knew of one other place. I don't remember the name of the pet store but it was on the outskirts of town. It was just a hole in the wall.

I told the owner I had a large dog with Displazia and he was sympathetic and produced a 100 ml bottle of Barbital which I purchased for about US$40.

I already have a test kit from Exit International which I will use when the time comes. The bottle, though, is sealed correctly, fresh from the factory. I will keep it in a cool, dry place until needed - if it is needed.

I cannot thank you enough for all of your help and your book. I am 83 years old and I live now with a great sense of relief.

Valladolid

Valladolid is a small city in Yucatán, about 2 hours drive from Cancun. Best known for its colonial architecture, especially its cathedral, the town is also used as a touring base for visiting the nearby Maya ruins.

Nembutal was first reported as being available over-the-counter in Valladolid back in 2010. Since then, other reports have emerged stating the same, but with some variations. In 2010, the cost of two bottles of Nembutal was 180 pesos each. In 2012 the price had risen to 600 pesos for two.

One store where Nembutal is available over-the-counter is Farmacia Veterinaria Los Potrillos at:

Calle 41 177-I
Col Valladolid Centro
Yucatan

At this animal pharmacy, the retail brand of Nembutal is Pisabental. Don't be surprised if the store does not have any bottles on the shelves. It is not uncommon for a store to send a messenger to the depot for collection. For the customer this may mean a return visit in an hour or two's time.

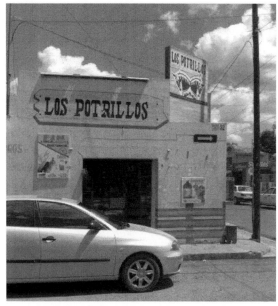

Fig 14.19: Farmacia Veterinaria Los Potrillos

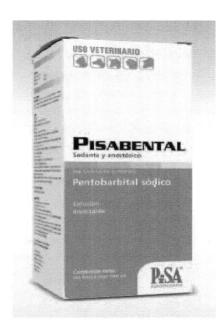

Fig 14.20: Pisabental: Mexican
sodium Pentobarbital

Tijuana

By late 2012, Nembutal was once again easily obtainable over-the-counter in Tijuana. This is not to say Tijuana is unchanged as a border city for it is very different from only a few years ago. Ten years ago, Tijuana was a bustling tourist destination. Five years ago it was a town wracked by drug war violence. At that time the very visible presence of the military made the city a frightening and intimidating place to visit. In 2012 Tijuana was reborn again. Its new face is worth noting.

In 2012 Tijuana was described as a ghost town but a very clean one at that. Gone were the soldiers with their machine guns. In their place is a visible, but not overwhelming, civilian police presence. Much the same as what you would find in US towns and cities anywhere. What is not visible is the tourist trade. Depsite streets so clean you could eat off them, there are scant tourisits around. In one way this is sad as the town has really cleaned up its act. The cheap tourist stores which line the Zona Centro around the main streest of Avenida Constitucion and Avenida Revolucion are still there but they are desperate for shoppers.

Another notable change in Tijuana is the dearth of vet stores. Whereas five years ago there was a vet store on every block. There are now only two farmacia veterinaria in operation. In addition to David's story of September 2012 following, Exit can report a second store in Del Travieso which is a pedestrian lane bordered by Av Constitucion and Revolucion and Benito Juarez y/o Segunda and Carillo Puerto (see the map in Fig 14.22). In 2013 a bottle of Pentobarbital at this veterinaria cost US$125, a considerable mark-up from the $45 it sold for in 2004.

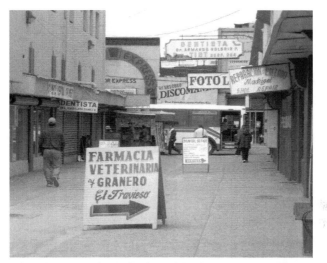

Fig 14.21a: Farmacia Veterinaria on El Travieso, Zona Centro Tijuana

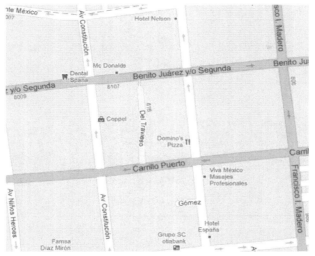

Fig 14.21b: Map featuring Farmacia Veterinaria on El Travieso

In 2012 David wrote:

> *I'd like to let you know that information in the PPeH has been very useful and I thank you.*
>
> *Last Wednesday I have been to Tijuana trying to buy Nembutal. I easily passed through the customs, walking . I crossed the two walking bridges and I immediately found a Vet. I asked for Anestesal, but the man told me that I needed a prescription. A little worried, I went to the very small store in Avenida Negrete suggested by your book. I asked for two bottles of Nembutal, I also showed the man in the store, who spoke good English, some photos from the book. He immediately gave me 2 bottles of Pentobarbital 100 ml. I paid $200. Done very easily. I was scared going back through the customs, but they didn't ask me anything. I bought a bottle of wiskey and a bottle of perfume, just to show that I bought something, I showed them and I passed through the scanner without problems.*
>
> *I hope my story can help someone, as I've been helped from your information.*

Other Cities in Mexico

In years gone by Nembutal has variously been available in Nuevo Progreso, Juarez, Nuevo Laredo, Nogales and Cancun. Exit has no knowledge of Nembutal ever being available in Reynosa, Del Rio or Matamoros.

Films taken of Laredo and Juarez in 2008-9 are included in this Chapter as background information only.

SOUTH AMERICA

Purchasing Nembutal in Person: Peru

For some years now, Exit has received reports confirming the ready, over-the-counter sale of veterinary Nembutal in Peru and Bolivia. Some positive accounts from Ecuador and Columbia have also been received, and these are being investigated.

In Peru, sodium pentobarbital is known by unique Peruvian names. The most common brand in this part of the world is 'Halatal'. A less common brand is called Penta. In Peru (unlike Mexico) Nembutal is sold in small 50ml bottles as opposed to 100ml bottles. However, the conctration is the same as that for the larger Mexican bottles. The concentration of both Halatal and Pento-Hypnol in Peru is 6.5gm per 100ml.

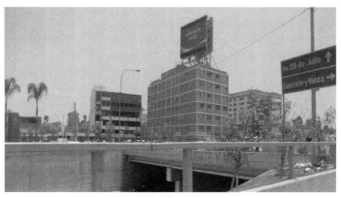

Fig 14.22: Suni Agro in Lima - Peru

Lima - Peru

As a sprawling capital city of 10 million, it is not surprising that Nembutal is easily available in Lima if one knows where to look. As in much of South America, it is the Agro-Veterinarias which readily sell Nembutal over-the-counter.

These stores differ from Mexican Farmacia Veterinaria in that they specialise in medicines and treatments for the rural sector and for farm animals, rather than domestic pets. Such stores are located all over Lima but one of the easiest to find is on a busy intersection adjacent to the 'Norte' (or northern) entrance of the 'Estadio Nacional' (national stadium), the home of the Peru national football team.

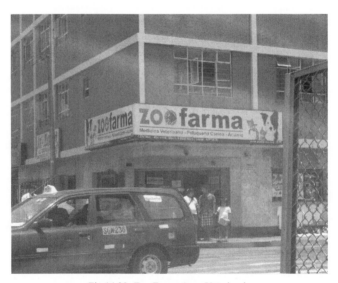

Fig 14.23: Zoo Farma Agro Veterinaria

Located at the intersection Santa Beatriz in central Lima, Zoo Farma is an Agro Veterinaria which takes 20-30 minutes by taxi ride from the popular tourist hotels of the Miraflores district, depending upon the traffic. (In Lima, taxis are relatively cheap with the average rate per hour costing between 25 and 30 Peruvian soles. Hotels routinely organise cabs for guests which is one way of guaranteeing guest safety for the inexperienced traveller).The entrance to Zoo Farma can be found at street level on the front corner of the large bright blue, six-story landmark building (see Fig 14.23), directly across the street from the stadium.

In 2013, a standard 50ml bottle of 'Halatal' at Zoo Farma retailed for 27 soles. The bottles are stored in the glass display cabinet under the counter, to the left of the entrance as one enters the store. To purchase Nembutal at Zoo Farma, simply ask for 'Halatal' (silent H) and the store attendant will oblige, issuing a receipt with your purchase.

In March 2013, Betty wrote to Exit with the following:

I booked a hotel in the Miraflores district of Lima, about a 55 Sol cab ride from the airport. This is a trendy, tourist-friendly, upscale area of town, close to the ocean with a busy shopping district. I then took a cab to the north entrance of the National Stadium as the book recommends (20 Sol), then entered the Zoo Farma (pictured adjacent page). They said they would not sell Halatal without a prescription, but suggested some of the neighboring shops would.

I then went door-to-door and one shop sold me four 50ml bottles of Halatal (the shop person sent their runner out to fetch them and was back in about 10 min). I paid 40 Sol each, 160 total at this location. I then tried another shop in

*the same vicinity and they had Pento-Hypnol in stock, but
would only sell me one 50ml bottle (the people at this shop
gave me a concerned look as I purchased it).*

*As the book mentions, there are vet med shops all over
Lima, but the location the book specifies has many shops in
a close proximity so it's best to start there.*

Cuzco - Peru

For those who are up for adventure, the UNESCO world herit-
age city of Cuzco makes for an easy shopping trip. An hour's
flight SE of Lima, the city of Cuzco is mostly known as the
jumping off point for visitors to the stunningly beautiful hidden Inca village of Machu Picchu. That Cuzco is also an extremely easy place to purchase Nembutal is a bonus.

In Cuzco, it is stores called 'Agro Veterinarias' which stock
Halatal (the only retail brand available). Exit has received
traveller reports that the Hotel Casa Andina is particularly
helpful in the purchase of Nembutal (organising a cab etc), but
travellers will likely find most hotels helpful.

The Agro Veterinarias in Cuzco are all quite close to the tourist area of the old colonial city. Depending on the location of
your hotel, (and one's ability to deal with the 3500m altitude of
Cuzco) it is possible to walk to these stores. In daylight hours,
this area of Cuzco is safe for tourists to stroll around. However, if you prefer to take a taxi, the hotel will call a trusted one
for you. The cost for the cab will be around 10 soles (~US$3)
which would include the 5 minutes wait time needed for you
to do your shopping.

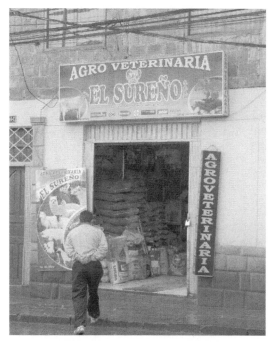

Fig 14.25: One of the many Agro Veterinarias in
Calle Tres Cruces de Oro in Cuzco, Peru

In Cuzco, an unremarkable street called 'Calle Tres Cruces de Oro' (the three golden crosses) is home to well over 10 veterinaras. Almost all of these Agro Veterinarias stock Halatal. Most stores have the boxes on open display either on the shelf behind or in front of the counter, or in a glass cabinet under the counter. In 2012 the cost of a single 50ml bottle of Halatal ranges between 22 and 25 soles (US$8-$9). It is advisable to purchase two - three bottles (6 - 9gm of Nembutal).

To purchase Halatal from any of the stores in these streets, one needs only to know the drug name, although a photo of a bottle can be useful. Spanish is not required as there will be no questions asked about what the drug is used for; the store attendants simply want to make a sale.

Stores which sell Nembutal (always called Halatal) in Calle Tres Cruces de Oro include:

- Casagroveto, El Progreso at No. 461
- Agroveterinaria Belen (Principal) at No. 496
- Progensa EIRL at No. 485
- Sucursal (Branch) at No: 421

In 2011, Jeff from Canada reported:

I just returned from a one week stay in Cuzco, Peru where I was successful in obtaining Halatal. The street Calles Tres Cruces has a long line of veterinary shops ... I went to Agroveterinaria ... There I got two fifty mL bottles for US $20.

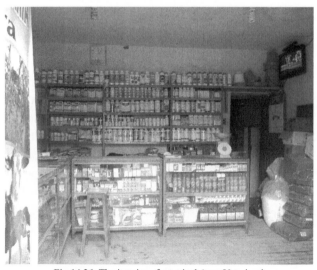

Fig 14.26: The interior of a typical Agro Veterinaria

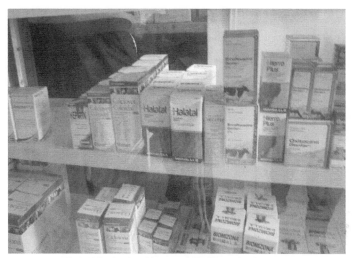

Fig 14.27: Nembutal boxes on display under the counter

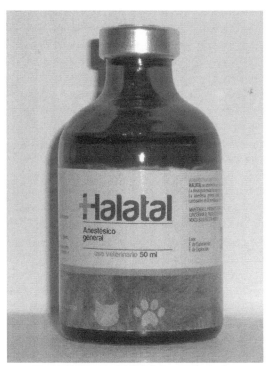

Fig 14.28: Peruvian Halatal in its new packaging

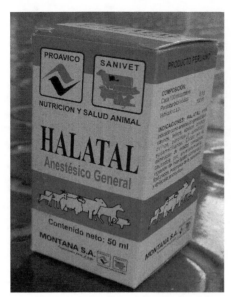

Fig 14.29: Peruvian veterinary sterile Nembutal:

Note - this packaging has been superseeded by that displayed in Fig 14.30

Fig 14.30: Peruvian veteri-nary sterile Nembutal:

Penta-Hypnol as it is occasionally retailed in Peru & Bolivia

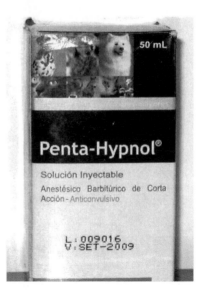

In 2012, Heather wrote:

After buying three bottles of Halatal at various stores in Calle Tres Cruces de Oro (and a marvellous visit on the Orient Express' Hiram Bingham to Machu Picchu), I was shocked to be stopped by police at Cusco airport on my way back to Lima.

As it turned out it was a random spot check. I was subject to a cursory going-through of my bags during which time they of course found my bottles of Nembutal. I was never asked what they were for, only if I had been sick from the altitude. When I nodded the bottles were carefully re-wrapped by the policeman in my sweater and that was that. I must say I was initially quite shocked to be singled out. Me - a drug runner - never. At least not the type of drugs they were looking for.

La Paz - Bolivia

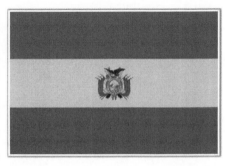

La Paz in Bolivia is the highest capital city in the world and, as such, its altitude may not suit all travellers. Like Cuzco, Nembutal is readily available in La Paz if you know what to ask for. In La Paz, Nembutal is sold under the trade name 'Halatal'. A cab ride to a local vet store should prove a simple way to make your purchase. If the store you visit does not have any in stock, they should offer to order it in.

To purchase Nembutal in Bolivia, you need no papers, no prescription, there are few reported complications. One traveller even had the vet offer to deliver his Nembutal order to his hotel. He paid US$10 for each 50ml bottle. Other travellers to this country have reported paying up to US$40 for a 100ml bottle. Either way, the price is appropriate and there is no sign of profiteering.

In La Paz, one pentobarbital is commonly sourced from the veterinary outlet at:

Av. Saavedra No 1004
Zona Miraflores, La Paz

SE ASIA

Since 2009, Exit has received many positive reports of the over-the-counter sale of Nembutal in Southeast Asia. However, as with South America, the availability of this drug seems to change with alarming frequency. What was true last month, is not true now.

Bangkok - Thailand

In 2011, reports of successful purchase of Nembutal over-the-counter from veterinary pharmacies in Bangkok ceased.

The Eieng Sew Tung Dispensary - on Ratchaprarop Road in Bangkok that had been a reliable source is now claiming it no longer sells Nembutal, not even to Thai nationals.

If you'd like to prove us wrong however, here are the details:

Eieng Sew Tung Dispensary
475/9 Ratchaprarop Rd,
Makkasan, Ratchatewee, Bangkok 10400
Tel : +66-2251-1482 Fax: +66-2251-7238

In the past travellers paid 850 Thai Baht (US$25) per 100 ml bottle. The retail name was Nembutal and the drug was manufactured by the French company CEVA.

Southern Thailand

Exit occasionally receives reports of the availability of liquid, veterinary Nembutal from veterinary stores in the town of Trang (near Phuket Island). The nearby town of Hat Yai (a larger town on the border of Malaysia) in Southern Thailand is one other noted possibility.

In both these towns, the liquid, veterinary Nembutal has been purchased from vet pharmacies/ hospitals. Both these towns are serviced by airports making access straight forward.

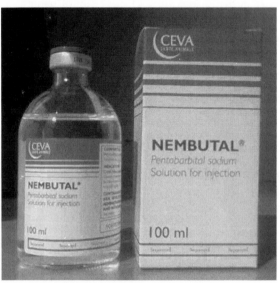

Fig 14.31: Sterile veterinary Nembutal as it is
retailed in Thailand

Concluding Comments

Nembutal continues to be sold over-the-counter and over the Internet from several countries around the world.

However, while the purchase of Nembutal might be quick and legal in some countries, the importation of Nembutal to your home country is *almost certainly illegal* and may attract penalties. You would nee to check the particular laws of the jurisdiction in which you reside to be certain.

However, if a seriously ill person purchases Nembutal lawfully in one country and then takes the drug and ends their life *in that country*, it is likely no laws will be broken.

15

Using Nembutal for a Peaceful Death

- Available forms of Nembutal
- Testing the sample before use
- Taking a sample for testing
- Opening the bottle of veterinary Nembutal
- Using the drug for a peaceful death
- Storage and Shelf life of Nembutal
- Interaction of Nembutal with other drugs
- Other useful barbiturates

Available forms of Nembutal

Since 2010, the availability of reagent grade sodium pentobarbital powder from Chinese manufacturers has meant that this form of the drug has superseded less readily available forms. (Fig 15.1)

For the past decade, sterile veterinary liquid has been the commonest form used for a peaceful death. (Fig 15.2)

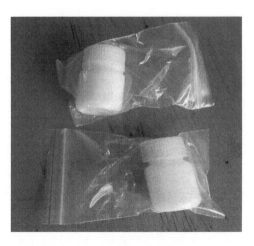

Fig 15.1: 25gm of Chinese powdered sodium pentobarbitol

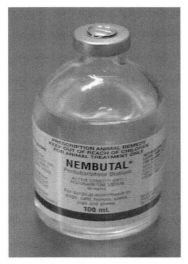

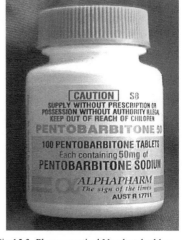

Fig 15.2: Sealed veterinary Nembutal   Fig 15.3: Pharmeceutical Nembutal tablets

Occasionally pharmaceutical grade Nembutal tablets or capsules, originally prescribed as sleeping medication, are obtained although this is uncommon. (Fig 15.3)

Reagent grade Nembutal is marketed as a white crystalline powder which readily absorbs moisture and is very soluble in water.

It is non sterile and packaged in small tightly sealed screw top plastic containers. Most people ordering in this way from China (see Ch 14) receive 25gm as loose powder packaged in a screw top plastic container (see Fig 15.1). Note that this is more than enough of the drug to provide a peaceful death for 2 - 3 people.

The veterinary liquid form of the drug is designed for intravenous administration in animals to provide anaesthesia for surgery. It is marketed as a sterile clear liquid with a concentration of 60 mg/ml of sodium pentobarbital in alkaline buffered solution with 10% methyl alcohol and ethylene glycol. The usual packaging is a glass 100ml bottle (clear or tinted glass), sealed with a rubber stopper and metal seal.

Pharmaceutical grade Nembutal tablets or capsules are normally supplied in a screw top plastic container, showing a date of manufacture of more than 20 years ago, usually long past their expiry date.

Testing the Sample Before Use

There are a number of reasons why one may wish to test the quality of their acquired Nembutal before using it for a peaceful death. For example, the drug may have come from a questionable source. Or it may have been kept for a number of years and may be the risk of significant deterioration. The question of reliability is of paramount importance. People do not want to take a substance if there is any question as to the outcome.

Taking a sample for testing

The tests described below require only a small sample of the powder or veterinary liquid to be tested (~ 0.5gm of powder or 6ml of veterinary liquid is enough to carry out all of the tests)

To use the Exit Spot Test for powdered Nembutal, use a clean knife to place a small sample of the powder on digital scales (see Fig 15.4).

A sample of veterinary liquid Nembutal for the Spot Test can be obtained as follows: The veterinary packaging is designed so that variable amounts of the drug can be withdrawn from the 100ml bottle using a syringe and hypodermic needle without breaking the sterile seal. Although there is no need for the Nembutal to be sterile, the drug keeps longer if the seal is not damaged and the solution remains sterile. The bottle should only be opened when the drug is either to be used or discarded. This is done by breaking the seal and removing the rubber stopper.

To take a small sample of the liquid for testing, remove the plastic cap from the tip of the bottle (if present) and then use a small knife or screwdriver to remove the small central circular metal piece covering the rubber stopper (Fig 15.5). This will expose the rubber seal. The needle of the hypodermic can then be pushed through the stopper into the bottle. Use the hypodermic 0.5ml syringe supplied with the Exit Nembutal Test Kit (or an equivalent). With the needle in place, invert the bottle and carefully withdraw the syringe plunger until there is 0.01ml of liquid in the syringe.

The testing process

Stage #1: Is the drug the barbiturate Nembutal?
This is often referred to as the <u>qualitative</u> 'Spot' test

Stage #2: Determining whether the Nembutal is pure, or has it deteriorated or been adulterated?
These are the <u>quantitative</u> tests. Several are discussed below.

a) Testing for water content
b) The melting point test
c) Purity testing using titration
d) Purity testing using gas chromatography

Stage #1: The Qualitative "Spot" Test using monoclonal antibodies

The Exit Spot Test Kit is an extremely useful screening test that can be quickly used if there is any doubt that Nembutal powder from China or liquid Nembutal from Peru or Mexico is, in fact, Nembutal. Only a very small sample is needed for the test (~0.1gm of powder, or 0.01ml of veterinary liquid). The Kit consists of a sealed dipcard and 0.5ml hypodermic syringe. (see Fig 15.8)

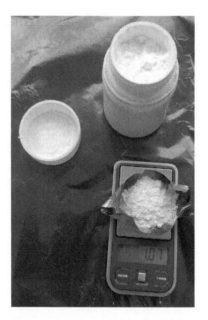

Fig 15.4: Weighing out Nembutal powder for testing

For veterinary liquid, use the syringe to remove a small sample from the bottle of drug to be tested using the method shown in Fig 15.5. Remove the dipcard from the foil pouch and remove the plastic cap to expose the absorbent tip. Saturate the absorbent tip of the dipcard with the veterinary liquid being tested and replace the plastic cap. Read the results of the test off the dipcard at 5 minutes. Do not interpret results after 10 minutes.

In the case of powdered product for testing, dissolve a small amount of powder in a few ml of distilled water. Saturate the absorbent tip of the dipcard and proceed as above.

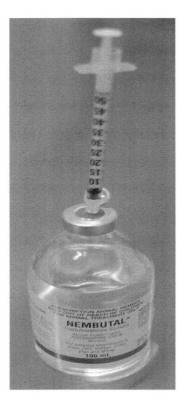
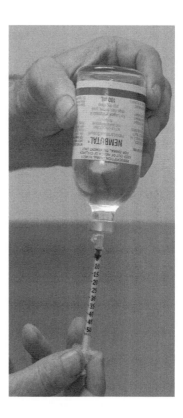

Fig 15.5: Removing a sample of Nembutal

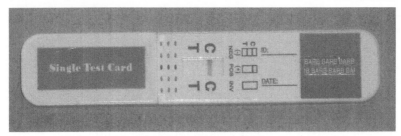

Fig 15..8 A positive 'Spot' Test

Reading the Test (Fig 15.8)
Negative Result: Two lines appear. A red line in the control region (C), and a red or pink line in the test region (T).

Positive: One red line in the control region (C). NO line appears in the test region (T). The absence of a test line indicates a positive result for Nembutal. Invalid: NO line appears in the control region (C).

Stage #2 Testing
a) Determining water content

The presence of water in any significant amount in a sample of Nembutal powder is an adverse finding. The power absorbs water from the air and must always be kept tightly sealed.

To determine water content, accurately weigh out ~1 gm of the powder and place in a laboratory oven with the temperature controlled at 100°C. After 30 minutes in the oven, let the powder cool in a desiccator and reweigh to establish the % water content. This should be < 5%

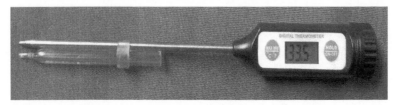

Fig 15.9: Digital thermometerwithglass meltingpoint capillary attached

b) The Melting Point Test

The Melting Point test is a useful test but it must be carried out on the free acid - not the sodium salt. Items needed for the test include a sealed glass capillary tube, thermometer (mercury or digital) with range > 150°C, and a glass container of cooking oil that can be heated slowly on the stove. (Fig 15.9)

If one has the powdered salt from China, or a bottle of liquid solution of the salt, the process is as follows: Take a sample (~0.5gm of the powder, or 3-5 ml of liquid, add a dilute acid (vinegar works well) to precipitate the free acid from solution, filter with a coffee filter paper then dry gently at ~ 100°C - 110°C. Place some of the dry pentobarbital crystals into the capillary and suspend in the oil. Heat the oil slowly on the stove and watch for the point at which melting of the crystals occurs. The crystals should change colour quickly from white to transparent at 131°C +/- 1°C.

A video of this process will be included in a future *eHandbook* update. A detailed description of the process with clear photographs has been posted on the Exit Forum by 'htveld'. This site can be visited in the Exit Forum 'Prime Posts' listing or see Fig 15.9a and Tab.   *http://bit.ly/HGv8tH*

c) Titration Testing

Reliable testing to quantify the presence of adulterants or degradation products requires sophisticated testing. A useful titration test can be carried out at home but it is important that careful attention to detail be followed to obtain reliable results. It is necessary to accurately weigh out a small sample of powder (~200mg +/- 0.5mg), dry in an oven at 100°C to determine the

Melting Point Test

Creating pentobarbital crystals

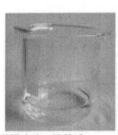
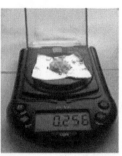
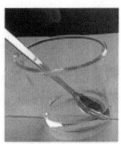

1) Fill a beaker with 30 mL of distilled water.

2) Weigh out approximately 250 mg of sodium pentobarbital powder.

3) Add the powder to the beaker and stir until dissolved.

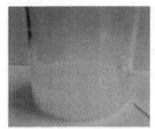
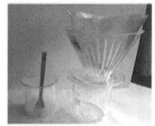

4) Add 9-10 mL of 0.1 M HCl solution to the beaker. The solution will become very cloudy. (you can also use 4 mL of white vinegar)

5) Pour the solution from the beaker into a coffee filter. Use some distilled water to wash out the residue.

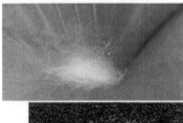
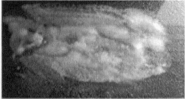
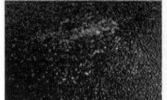
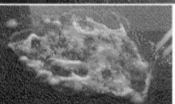

6) Leave to dry for a while, then thinly spread out the residue in the filter on a plate. Let it dry for 24 hours at room temperature, or in an oven at 100 degrees Celcius.

The residue may look like any of the above images.

Fig 15.9a: Step by Step test of Nembutal Purity using Melting Point Test by 'htveld' @ Exit Forum

Gas Chromatography Analytical Results

Specimen Code	Specimen Type	Pentobarbital-Na % w/w	Loss on Drying % w/w
A	White Powder	95.2	2.5
B	White Powder	96.2	1.8
C	White Powder	95.2	3.2
D	White Powder	95.0	2.6
E	White Powder	95.2	2.4
F	White Powder	95.6	2.7
G	White Powder	96.0	1.9

Certificate of Analysis

Product Name	Pentobarbital sodium/57-33-0 reagent grade		
Batch No.	20100409	Quantity	200g
Date of Production	20100409	Expiry Date	20120409
Product standard	In-house standard		

Item	Requirements	Test Results
Description	White crystalline powder	Complies
Solubility in Water	Easy soluble	Complies
Assay	≥98.0%	99.1%
Conclusion	Meets the Requirements	

Fig 15.10: GC Analysis of 4 Chinese samples along with sample 'B' Analysis certificate

Endpoint in sodium pentobarbital titration:

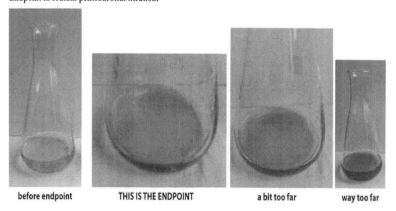

before endpoint   THIS IS THE ENDPOINT   a bit too far   way too far

Fig 15.10a: Methyl Orange titration for Nembutal purity by 'htveld'

presence of any significant amount of water in the specimen, then titrate with hydrochloric acid, using methyl orange as an indicator.

A detailed step by step account of this process has been provided to Exit by 'htveld' and is available on the 'Prime Posts' section of the Exit Forum (or see Tab). *http://bit.ly/HGv8tH*

d) Purity using Gas Chromatography

The gold standard for testing the purity of a sample is to carry out testing with gas chromatography. The necessary equipment needed to carry out such tests restrict this to commercial laboratories. The Exit laboratory operates such equipment (see Fig 16.7) and uses it to calibrate the other easier methods.

Exit has been able to test a number of samples of Nembutal sourced from China and Mexico using Gas Chromatography and has seen no evidence of significant adulteration or deterioration, even in samples that have been stored for long periods (some over 15 years). Recent test runs have looked at seven powder Nembutal samples from different Chinese sources, all delivered purity results >95%. The results for the seven analysis and the Analysis Certificate accompanying one of the samples is shown (see Fig 15.10). Chinese suppliers who have had samples tested by Exit are listed with an '*' (see Chapter 14)

Nembutal Testing

In 2013, Exit launched a home Dilution-Purity Test Kit (Quantitative test). This is available from: *http://www.exitinternationalstore.com/Exit-Dilution-Purity-Test-Kit-quantitative-BARB-TEST-QUAN.htm*

Australian members of Exit also have the benefit of a mobile testing facility. Exit does not take possession of the substances tested. Ownership remains with the person carrying out the tests. An extension of this program to other countries is under consideration.

Storage and Shelf Life of the Barbiturates

The soluble barbiturate salts (viz pentobarbital sodium) are very stable drugs, and if stored correctly maintain their potency for decades. This is a particularly useful property of Nembutal, as it means the drug can be obtained and safely stored many years before any potential use.

In powdered form, sodium pentobarbital should be kept tightly sealed away from any contamination or exposure to oxygen or atmospheric moisture. The product from China is usually supplied loosely packed in a small plastic sachet, so re-packaging is important. There are two recommended procedures for long term storage.

Method #1: Find a suitable glass container with a airtight screw top. The size should just accommodate the powder, with little extra space for air. If testing is planned, remove ~500mg, then tightly seal the container before wrapping it in aluminium foil (to protect from the light) and store it in a cool place. The refrigerator (~4^{0}C is fine). Do not freeze.

Method #2: (Courtesy of Alan Davies) An alternative strategy is to wrap the sample (minus 500mg if testing is planned) in aluminium foil, and place the package in a metallized Mylar (PET) bag. The bag is then vacuum sealed using a home vacuum food storage unit (such as the Sunbeam VS780 'Food Saver')

Fig 15.10c Stages in vacuum packaging powdered Nembutal

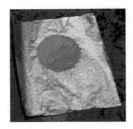   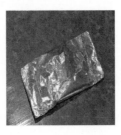   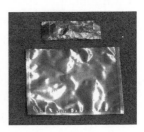

10gm of powder in foil   Powder wrapped in foil   Place in Mylar storage bag

Silica Gel
moisture
absorbing
sachet

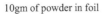

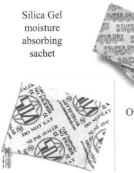

O^2 absorbing
sachet

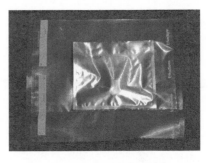

Place the vacuum sealed Mylar bag
inside a PE 'Food Saver' bag

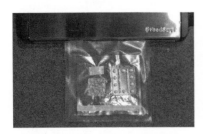

Above: Vacuum seal the Mylar bag
inside a plastic PE bag along with
moisture and oxygen absorbing sachets

Right: The finished package ready for
storage

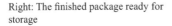

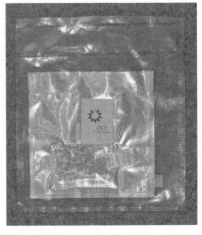

15cm x15cm Mylar bags are ideal and provide ideal oxygen and moisture protection to the sample. The sealed Mylar bag is itself then vacuum packed inside a standard polyethylene food serve bag (~25cm x 20cm), along with moisture (silica gel) and oxygen absorbing sachets. The finished sample is small can then be conveniently stored in a cool place (< 20⁰C).

Any indication that the seal is broken is obvious as the package becomes pliable, at which point the outer vacuum package can be replaced.

Note: Extracting all the air from Mylar bags before heat sealing an sometimes prove difficult because of the smooth finish of the bag. A solution to this is shown on YouTube
Vacuum Seal Mylar bags - Problem Solved
http://www.youtube.com/watch?v=r9dzaeC0hG0

Note: Moisture and oxygen absorbing sachets and Mylar bags are available at small cost on the internet. See for example:
https://www.usaemergencysupply.com/

Note: Some have suggested including 6 x 10mg metoclopramide anti-emetic tablets along with the sachets before the final vacuum seal. However it is NOT clear that the shelf life of the anti-emetic would be increase with this storage method.

Veterinary liquid comes in sealed sterile glass 100ml containers and should be left undisturbed until it is to be needed. Do not break the seal and decant the liquid into another container as this will expose the drug to the air. Store the bottles in a cool dark place. Refrigeration is fine but again do not freeze. The liquid should be clear and colourless. Any colouration or precipitation after long storage periods indicates that testing and assay is necessary.

Pharmaceutical grade Nembutal capsules or tablets are likely to have deteriorated because of their age and should be tested before use.

Note: Previous editions of the Peaceful Pill eHandbook outlined a method of long term storage that involved the conversion of the salt (sodium pentobarbital, CAS No 57-33-0) to the free acid (pentabarbital CAS No 76-74-4). The success of vacuum packing the salt has led to the removal of this method from the main text, but the information is still included as a Tab on this page for those who are interested.

Interaction with Other Drugs

Those who take Nembutal for a peaceful death are often taking other drugs for various health problems. When approaching the chosen time to take the Nembutal, the question is often asked about whether any intercurrent medications should cease.

There are few drugs that interfere significantly with the action of Nembutal, making it less effective. This is why there is no absolute need to cease taking other drugs in the preceding days. However, it is common for those planning their death to cease all but the essential medication in the week before their planned exit.

There is some evidence that chronic heavy alcohol use may lead to cross-tolerance and significantly impair the action of the barbiturate. Another instance would be the rare case where someone has been taking another barbiturate for some time and has developed a barbiturate-tolerance in this way. This is uncommon although occasionally people take the anti-

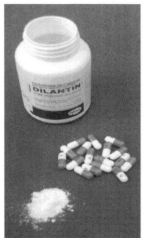

Fig 15.11: Dilantin 100mg capsules

convulsant barbiturate, phenobarbital, for long periods. In these cases, a larger dose of the Nembutal (12gm powder or 2 x 100ml bottles) would be advised.

Some drugs enhance the effect of the Nembutal and can even be employed for that specific purpose. An example is the anti-convulsant Dilantin (phenytoin sodium Fig 15.11).

Dilantin is useful as the drug dissolves in water forming an alkali solution which is compatible with the liquid Nembutal. If you have a bottle of Nembutal which is of uncertain quality, the potency can be enhanced by dissolving 1- 2gm of phenytoin sodium in the liquid Nembutal before drinking. This process is shown in the accompanying video 'Making Nembutal even more effective'.

Although Dilantin is a drug that is controlled, it is relatively easily obtained through Internet mailing sources. It is not a drug that attracts attention.

Other Useful Barbiturates

Two other barbiturates that still find wide (although decreasing) use in medicine can also be usefully employed for a peaceful death. These are the anti-convulsant Phenobarbital, and the anaesthetic induction agent Pentothal.

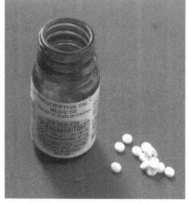

Fig 15.12: 30mg tablets of Phenobarbitone

Phenobarbital

As discussed in Chapter 13, phenobarbital and pentobarbital are drugs that are often confused because of the similarity of their names. Although both are barbiturates, pentobarbital sodium (Nembutal) is the fast-acting soluble salt. This is the euthanasia drug of choice in all countries that allow assisted suicide and euthanasia. Phenobarb is a different drug. In its usual form phenobarb is a slow-acting anti-convulsant, prescribed when there is a risk of convulsions (eg. brain trauma etc).

Some people will have access to phenobarb, either from their own doctor or from overseas pharmaceutical suppliers. 10gm (~ 250 of the white 30mg tablets shown in Fig 15.12) of crushed which is then mixed with water and taken as a drink will be lethal.

Note: There is no rapid loss of consciousness, as in the case of Nembutal. The time to death using phenobarbitone can be several hours. If one is found before death, resuscitation is very possible.

Phenobarb can, however, be made more effective by forcing up the pH of the solution of the crushed tablets. This is done using Sodium Carbonate to convert the Phenobarbital to the more readily-absorbed sodium phenobarbital. If available, 1gm of Dilantin can be added to this drink with good effect.

To reduce the time from taking the drink to loss of consciousness, a second drink made from a benzodiazepam sleeping drug is recommended (eg, Serapax, oxazepam or Mogadon, nitrazepam). Again, alcohol can be an effective supplement.

Pentothal (thiopentone sodium)

For many years, Pentothal was the main intravenous induction agent used in anaesthesia. Its use has declined in recent years. When given intravenously, most patients are asked by the anaesthetist to count back from 10. Few get past 7 before consciousness is lost.

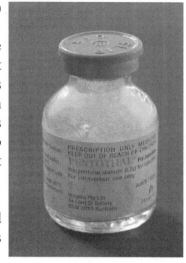

Note: This is the primary drug used in lethal injections in executions in the US. In November 2010, a worldwide shortage of the drug

Fig 15.13 500mg ampoule of dry Pentothal

prompted the state of Oklahoma to investigate using Nembutal as an alternative. See: *http://abcn.ws/dPu2Zr*

Pentothal is marketed as a soluble thiopentone sodium powder in sterile ampoules. These are designed to be mixed with sterile water before being administered intravenously.

The powder can be dissolved in water and taken with rapid effect orally. 10gm of the drug (the contents of 20 ampoules) dissolves rapidly in ~50ml of water, and if drunk leads to rapid loss of consciousness and death. Alcohol is a useful supplement.

Exit has looked at vacuum-packing 10gm of dry sodium pentothal powder mixed with 1gm of phenytoin sodium. This can be readily transported and stored.

Reconstitution is carried out by breaking the vacuum seal and dissolving the sachet of powder in ~50ml of water before drinking.

Concluding Comment

When rigorous scientific processes are used to establish the purity and efficacy of known drugs, thus ensuring a reliable and peaceful death, the need for legislative change is significantly diminished.   This is because the act of dying well and at a time and place of one's choosing is in reach of those who seek it, as long as certainly steps are taken. This not only removes the dying process from the hands of the medical profession but empowers the elderly and the seriously ill to make their own end-of-life decisions, should the need ever arise.

Whether legislation that provides controlled access to assistance to die exists or not, it is unlikely to effect the person who has their Peaceful Pill locked in the cupboard. When the time is right, they will simply go to the cupboard!

Is one 100ml bottle of veterinary Nembutal enough for a peaceful death?

While there are several florid accounts of failure by people taking a full 100ml bottle of veterinary Nembutal, closer scrutiny shows a much more complex situation. Exit has examined the details and medical records of several such cases.

In the vast majority of cases, one bottle (100ml @ 60mg/ml) of veterinary Nembutal will always be satisfactory. However, there is a small group (estimated at <1%) who may exhibit a prolonged comatose phase before death (sometimes up to 24 hours). Outright 'failures' remain extremely rare. Indeed, all of the reported failures investigated were associated with discovery and medical intervention. This emphasises the need for careful selection of the place of death.

In some of the analysed cases, the long comatose phase is associated with the prolonged use of anti-psychotic medication or chronic heavy alcohol use, prior to taking the barbiturate. It is presumed the induction of liver enzymes by these drugs causes increased degradation of the Nembutal, lowering the concentration in the brain. In these situations, increasing the quantity of drug taken (eg. to 2 bottles, 12gm) may not necessarily hasten the death.

Exit has examined the use of several potentiating drugs which may be dissolved into the liquid Nembutal, removing any possibility of extended coma. The most useful, Dilantin, (phenytoin sodium) is discussed in this Chapter.

Should one eat a meal before taking Nembutal?

The chance of reflex vomiting brought on by drinking the bitter Nembutal liquid is reduced if there is something in the stomach. This should not be a significant meal that will slow the absorption of the drug. Something light is preferable, like tea and toast, an hour or so before taking the drug.

 Is there something that can be added to the Nembutal liquid to take away the bitter taste?

It is always better to take one's Nembutal straight. The likely result of mixing the Nembutal with something else (eg. yogurt) is the creation of a greater volume of something equally unpalatable. Furthermore, using a spoon to consume the drug, rather than drinking it, can mean a longer time to ingest the 100ml. Exit has received reports of people falling asleep before all of the drug is consumed. This is dangerous. It is best to drink the 100ml in a few swallows, then drink alcohol.

16

The Peaceful Pill

Developing a Peaceful Pill

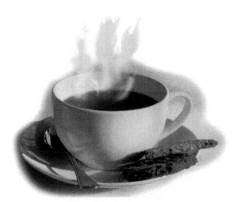

The ongoing difficulties in obtaining the best euthanasia drug, Nembutal has prompted Exit to establish an ambitious research project - the synthesis of one's own 'Peaceful Pill'.

The Peaceful Pill Project has run for several years. Many strategies have been explored and rejected with some significant advances made. In this Chapter we detail this Exit research and discuss in more detail the use of the drug Nembutal for a peaceful death.

The synthesis of a barbiturate-like pill, involves the acquisition of restricted and hard-to-get chemicals and the use of processes that are difficult and occasionally dangerous for the novice. Nevertheless, as the pathways are established and simplified, safer processes are developed and recorded. An outline of the steps required for barbiturate synthesis and assay are described and illustrated where possible with video.

The Nicky Finn

Exit's first trials of the home-made Peaceful Pill – the 'Nicky Finn' - were completed in 2004. Named after the famous Micky Finn drink of the Lone Star Saloon in Chicago in the early 1900s, Exit's Nicky Finn was made from alcohol and nicotine.

Manufactured by chlorinating alcohol and combining this chloral hydrate with pure nicotine, the Nicky Finn should prove highly effective and highly lethal when taken as a drink. Although synthesis was straightforward, the difficulty in testing this untried product left questions about this strategy unanswered.

Changing Focus

Exit International launched the 'Peanut Project' in early 2005. Named after an old-fashioned street term for barbiturate (Peanuts), the Peanut Project brought together a group of elderly people to create their own barbiturate. Could they synthesise Nembutal?

How could they make something that:

• they could take orally
• could be manufactured without outside assistance
• would provide a peaceful and dignified death
• would be reliable with negligible risk of failure.

The first Workshop was held in late 2005 on a remote property in the Australian countryside. The average age of participants was 80 years, although some were in their 90s. Several who participated were seriously ill.

Legal Issues

Setting out to manufacture one's own barbiturate Peaceful Pill exposes those involved to significant legal risk. In Australia, the manufacture of barbiturates is governed by laws such as the *Drug Misuse and Trafficking Act 1985 (NSW)* which makes it a crime to manufacture, possess or supply such a drug. The penalties that apply depend upon the amount of the prohibited drug involved. If the amount is less than 10gm, the penalty is two years jail and a fine of $5,500. If amounts greater than 20Kg are involved, the penalty is life in jail and a fine of $550,000.

In most western countries there will also be other laws that make it an offence to manufacture, possess, sell, supply and import certain narcotic and psychotropic drugs. Penalties will depend upon the amount of the drug involved, and again range from two years jail and a fine, to life imprisonment. Finally, there is the other additional generic legal question. If one member of the group ever took the substance the group made and died, would the remaining members be accused of having assisted with that person's suicide?

It was stated clearly at the start, that no one in the initial group would make more than they needed for themselves. No one was making a Pill for someone else, and no one would sell any of the substance manufactured. Finally, no one would acquire more than 10gm of the manufactured barbiturate (the common lethal dose) and any excess would be destroyed.

The first Peanut stage failed when a group member became disenchanted with the project and denounced those involved. Threats were made to inform the authorities of the group's activities and the project was forced to close for several years. The death of the member in 2010 led to the project's reestablishment in 2011.

The Chemistry

The processes used for the barbiturate Peaceful Pill synthesis have been known for many years. Barbiturates are derivatives of barbituric acid. which was first synthesised by Adolph von Bayer in 1864, by condensing malonic acid with urea.

An easier method makes use of the di-ethyl ester of malonic acid (di-ethyl malonate) which reacts with urea in the presence of a catalyst sodium ethoxide; a base is formed by dissolving metallic sodium in absolute alcohol (ethanol).

This synthesis can be depicted as follows.

Di-Ethyl Malonate   +   Urea   + (Sodium Ethoxide) =   Barbituric Acid

The reaction takes place under reflux for a number of hours at 110^0C. Crystals of barbituric acid are obtained by acidifying the reaction mixture, then filtering and cooling the filtrate. Barbituric acid, however, has no physiological activity. The process needs to be taken further to develop a barbiturate that can peacefully end life. The sedative, hypnotic, and anaesthetic properties of the barbiturates are determined by the characteristics of two additional side-arms (or side-chains) attached to the barbituric acid molecule.

The di-substituted barbiturates of particular interest are amylobarbital (Amytal) and pentobarbital (Nembutal). The process of adding side-arms (di-substitution) needs to be undertaken before the condensation of the malonate and urea.

In Amytal, the two alkyl side arms are (a) ethyl, introduced as ethyl-bromide and (b) 3-methylbutyl, introduced as 1-bromo-3-methylbutane. In Nembutal, the two alkyl side-arms are (a) ethyl, introduced as ethyl-bromide and (b) 1-methylbutyl, produced from 2-bromopentane. In both substitution reactions the malonate is heated, either in a closed pressure system (autoclave) or under reflux first with one and then the second alkyl bromide. In both reactions sodium ethoxide is used as the catalyst.

The final step in the production of sodium pentobarbital or sodium amylobarbital is heating of the resultant di-substituted malonate with dry urea in an autoclave or under reflux for another 12 hours. This is again done in the presence of dry alcohol and sodium. Excess alcohol is removed by distillation and the residue - predominantly sodium pentobarbital, or sodium amylobarbital - is dissolved in water to form the Peaceful Pill.

In all of the di-substitution reactions and in the condensation with urea, it is essential that there be absolutely no water present. Care must be taken to ensure no atmospheric moisture reaches the autoclave or reactor vessel. All substances used must be dry. In particular, the alcohol used in the production of the sodium ethoxide needs to be as dry as possible (super dry).

Equipment

In the original project, the period of prolonged reflux was carried out using a two-litre glass reaction vessel with three Quickfit taper necks (24/29), fitted with an efficient double surface condenser (Fig 16.1). A heating mantle and a means of stirring the mixture and monitoring the temperature were also required. To protect the reacting substances from atmospheric moisture, calcium chloride guard tubes were used. To remove excess alcohol in the final stage, the double-surface condenser was attached to the reactor vessel by means of a distillation head. The alcohol that was distilled was collected in a glass receiving vessel that was also fitted with a calcium chloride guard tube (Fig 16.5). An accurate chemical balance, capable of measuring to 0.1g, was required to weigh out the necessary reactants.

In the subsequent 'Single Shot' project, a specialised stainless steel pressurised reaction vessel (autoclave) was employed. This replaced the glassware and the reflux condenser. This sealed stainless steel vessel (autoclave) allowed the reaction to take place under pressure, shortened reaction time and reduced the problem of contamination from atmospheric moisture (Fig 16.2). Pressure was read directly from the gauge with the temperature in the reaction vessel read via a thermocouple (with an infrared thermometer used as backup).

To remove the substituted malonates from the reaction vessel a condenser was employed. This was made from stainless steel tubing surrounded by a water jacket. Connected to a receiving vessel of stainless steel this was then vented using a calcium chloride guard tube and placed under reduced pressure in the distillation process using a water tap vacuum attachment.

The setup of the glassware for reflux used is shown in Fig 16.1. Note: the presence of the guard tube on the top of the reflux condenser. The distillation setup is shown in Fig 16.3.

The single shot equipment is shown in Fig 16.2. The distillation set-up shown in Fig 16.4

Special Dangers

As with all chemical processes, care and attention to detail was needed at all times. The equipment was clean and dry before use. Many of the liquids used in the synthesis were flammable and naked flames were not used. Heating of the reaction vessel was by way of an electric hotplate. The most dangerous substances used in the process were metallic sodium and the strongly basic intermediary sodium ethoxide. Standard organic chemistry texts (eg. Solomons & Fryhle, 2004) spell out the dangers of handling these substances.

CAUTION: Sodium must be handled with great care and under no circumstances should the metal be allowed to come into contact with water as an explosion and fire may result. Sodium is stored under paraffin or xylene and should only be handled with tongs or tweezers, not with fingers.

Small waste or scrap pieces of sodium can be disposed of by placing them in a bottle containing large quantities of methylated spirits.

The commercial sodium is covered with a non-metallic crust. A sodium press can be constructed to remove this and produce clean sodium wire for the reaction vessel. See 'Betty cooks with Sodium' Fig 16.6).

Precursors

The list of necessary precursors (with their Chemical Abstract Service number, 'CAS No.') includes the following:

Di-ethyl malonate
CAS No: 105-53-3

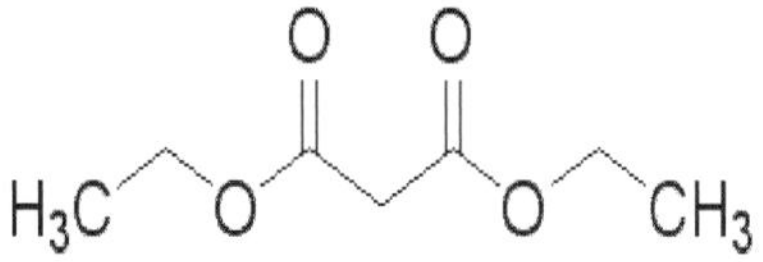

Alkyl sidechains:

a) Ethyl bromide
CAS No: 74-96-4

$$CH_3CH_2Br$$

and

b) 1-bromo-3-methylbutane
CAS No: 107-82-4 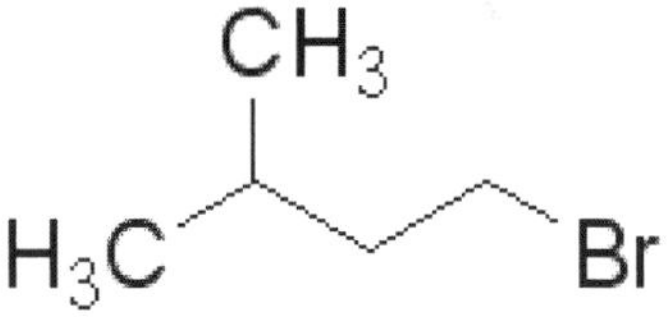
or
c) 2 Bromo-pentane
CAS No: 107-81-3

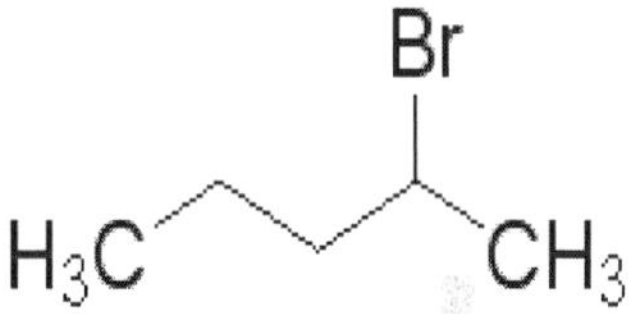

Catalyst
Sodium ethoxide
CAS No: 141-52-6

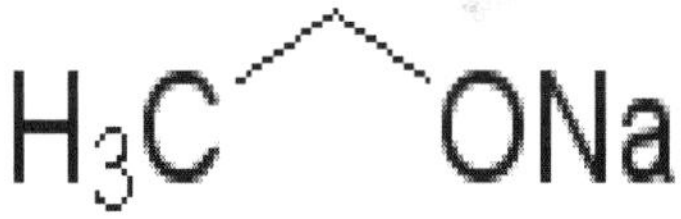

or

Sodium metal
CAS No: 7440-23-5
&
Absolute alcohol
CAS No: 64-17-5

Urea
CAS No: 57-13-6

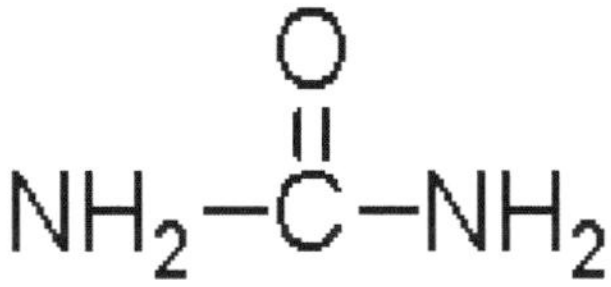

$$NH_2-\overset{O}{\underset{\|}{C}}-NH_2$$

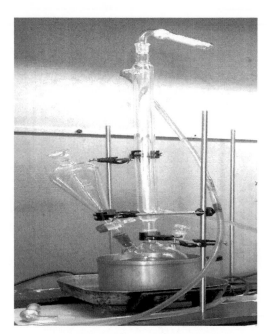

Fig 16.1: Reflux system
used for barbiturate
synthesis

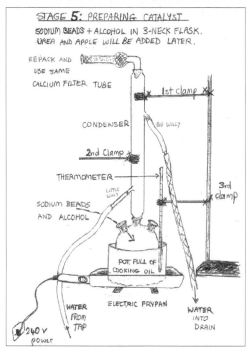

None of the chemicals required are subject to specific government restriction. Application to a reputable chemical supplier for ethyl malonate and the chosen side-chain alkyl bromides is generally successful provided one can detail a legitimate purpose in the required end-user statement. Some endeavour may be required to obtain the sodium metal and dry ethyl alcohol. Alternatively, the catalyst sodium ethoxide can be purchased.

Authors' note - the chemicals required to make a Peaceful Pill may be classified as 'precursors' for the synthesis of a restricted substance. Possession of significant quantities of these items may be an indictable offence and could result in significant penalties.

Acquiring Necessary Equipment

Laboratory glassware is becoming increasingly hard to obtain. This is a reaction on the part of the authorities to the existence of clandestine laboratories that manufacture illegal drugs (predominantly amphetamines) for commercial gain. The award-winning TV series 'Breaking Bad' is an excellent example of what can occur in the dark underworld of blackmarket drugs. Some of the chemical techniques used in the synthesis of a Peaceful Pill are the same as those used to make illicit drugs.

The synthesis in Exit's projects required a prolonged period of reflux (Fig 16.1). A glass reaction vessel with 3 Quickfit taper necks (24/29), fitted with an efficient double surface condenser was needed. A heating mantle and a means of stirring the mixture and monitoring the temperature were also used. To protect the reacting substances from atmospheric moisture calcium chloride guard tubes are needed. The double surface condenser can be attached to the reactor vessel by means of a distillation head.

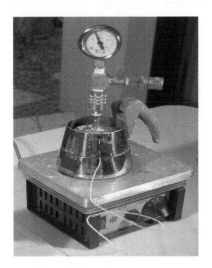

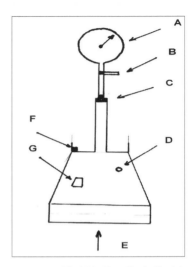

Fig 16.2: The 'Single Shot' Autovclave
A: Pressure Gauge
B: Distillation coupling
C: Pressure coupling
D: Pressure safety valve
E: Heat + Stirring
F: Thermocouple
G: IR thermometer patch

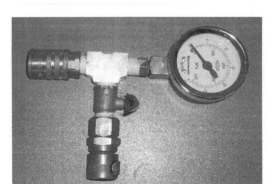

Fig 16.3: Autoclave pressure head

Fig 16.4: Vacuum distillation setup
A: Autoclave
B: Heat + Stirring
C: Condenser water jacket
D: Calcium chloride guard tube
E: Vacuum line
F: Collection vessel

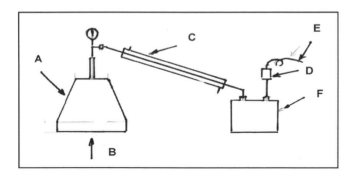

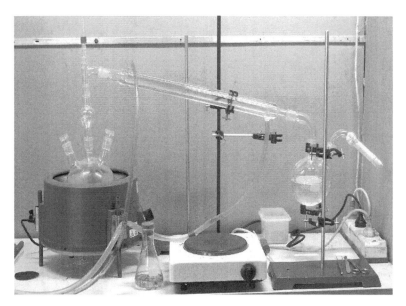

Fig 16.5: Glass distillation system

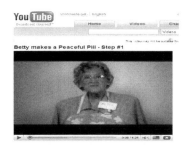

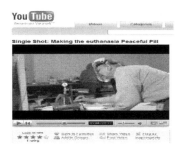

Fig 16.6: Single Shot on *YouTube*

A glass receiving vessel, fitted with a calcium chloride guard tube, is needed to collect the distillate (Fig 16.5).

An accurate chemical balance capable of measuring to 0.1g is required in order to weigh out the necessary reactants.

Distributors of this specialized glassware (eg. reaction vessels with Quickfit necks, double-surface condensers, distillation heads, guard tubes etc) are often required to inform authorities of 'suspicious' purchases. For this reason it can be helpful to know someone who has access to laboratory glassware and glass-blowing skills.

The manufacture of specialised equipment in stainless steel avoids some of these difficulties. The stainless reaction autoclave used in the 'Single Shot' process has been adapted from a coffee pot. This method has since been modified as problems with the process were realised. The equipment now used consists of:

- a stainless steel pressure reactor vessel with pressure and temperature monitor and stirring facility
- a stainless condenser used for reflux and solvent extraction
- a stainless receiving container fitted with calcium chloride guard tubes

Stages in Barbiturate Synthesis

There are three basic steps in the synthesis of a barbiturate Peaceful Pill:

- Step 1: Attaching the first sidechain to the di-ethyl malonate
- Step 2: Attaching the second sidechain to the product of step 1
- Step 3: Condensing the di-substituted malonate with urea to form the required barbiturate

Looking at these steps in more detail

Step 1

In the case of the target barbiturates, Nembutal or Amytal, the first sidechain to be attached to the di-ethyl malonate is an ethyl halide, usually ethyl bromide is used. To form the mono-sustituted malonic ester, ethyl bromide is heated with the di-ethyl malonate in the presence of the required catalyst - the base, sodium ethoxide.

The catalyst may be purchased or made as part of the process. To make the required ethoxide add 5.7g of metallic sodium that has been cleaned by passing through a press - see 'Betty cooks with Sodium' - and 125ml of very dry alcohol.

Into this mixture of dry alcohol and sodium ethoxide add 38ml of di-ethyl malonate and 26g of bromoethane. Heat is applied and the mixture stirred using a magnetic stirrer. In an open system a reflux condenser must be fitted and a calcium chloride guard tube used to ensure no contamination by atmospheric moisture.

Note: Super Dry Alcohol

Alcohol (ethanol) of the required dryness can be made using methylated spirits as the starting point (95.6% alcohol). Absolute ethanol (>99.5%) is obtained by heating this under reflux with dry (recently fired) calcium oxide. To significantly improve the yield in the synthesis of barbiturates, even dryer alcohol is required. To remove more of the water, thereby converting the 99.5% ethanol to 'super dry' alcohol (>99.8%), use 5gm of magnesium turnings with 0.5gm of iodine in a boiling vessel. Let the magnesium react with ~50ml of the 99.5% ethanol producing hydrogen and magnesium ethanolate. When all of the magnesium has been consumed, the remainder of the absolute alcohol is added, refluxed for 30 minutes, and distilled directly into the planned storage vessel. The resulting ethanol should be better than 99.95%. See the Video 'Making super dry alcohol'.

Step 2
Sodium ethoxide catalyst is again needed in the reaction vessel, and this time 47g of the monosubstituted ester from Step 1 is converted to a di-substituted ester by reflux (or reaction in an autoclave) with the second side chain. For the synthesis of Amytal, this second sidechain is 1-bromo-3 methylbutane. In the case of Nembutal, it is 2-bromopentane, in each case 38g is required.

At the end of this stage the di-substituted malonate is removed again by vacuum distillation. This is 3-methyl-butyl-ethyl malonic ester in the case of Amytal synthesis; 1-methyl butyl-ethyl malonic ester if Nembutal is being manufactured.

Step 3
Sodium ethoxide is again needed in the reaction vessel. For this final step 58g of the di-substituted malonate from step 2 is allowed to react with 15g of dry urea that has been dissolved in hot dry alcohol. The mixture is stirred and heated under reflux. After 4 hours, the excess alcohol is boiled off and the residue dissolved in water and acidified (with dilute hydrochloric acid) to precipitate the insoluble barbiturate crystals which can be washed and dried.

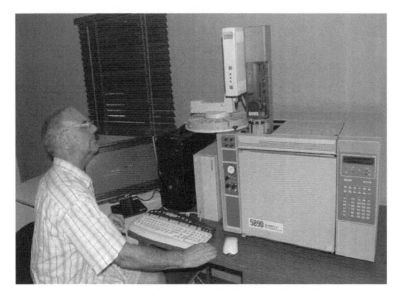

Fig 16.7: Exit gas chromatography equipment

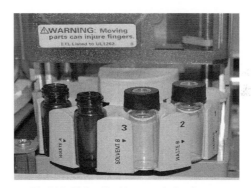

Fig 16.8: Vials of barbiturate solution for assay

Testing the Product

As with any home-made product, careful testing is necessary. The best method for this is using gas chromatography and mass spectroscopy (GC-MS).

For those who do not have access to such sophisticated laboratory equipment - and lets face it - that is most folk - Exit sells both a qualitative and quantitative test kit at our online store at: www.exitinternationalstore.com

Detailed instructions on the use of the full range of Nembutal purity test is published on an ongoing basis as updates in the online *Peaceful Pill eHandbook*.

17

The Swiss Option

Introduction

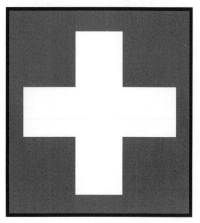

There is only a handful of places in the world where Voluntary Euthanasia and/ or Assisted Suicide is currently legal.

In those US States that have assisted suicide, citizens and residents who qualify can obtain a prescription for the lethal drug Nembutal. In these states, however, a doctor cannot provide more assistance than this, with voluntary euthanasia remaining illegal. It is solely Physician Assisted Dying (PAD) or Physician Assisted Suicide that is legal (see *Killing Me Softly: VE and the Road to the Peaceful Pill* for more discussion of the difference between VE, PAD or PAS).

To make use of Oregon or Washington's Death with Dignity laws, however, a person must be a resident of that state and be able prove this with suitable documents. It is not enough to be a Californian. Rather, the law is only open to 'true' Oregonians and Washingtonians respectively.

In the Netherlands, the *Termination of Life on Request and Assisted Suicide Act 2002* allows voluntary euthanasia, but there are strict residential requirements. In this country, a person wanting to make use of the law must satisfy medical requirements and have a *long-standing relationship with a Dutch doctor.* This effectively restricts the use of this euthanasia law to Dutch citizens.

In Belgium and Luxemburg, where voluntary euthanasia was legalized in 2002 and 2009 respectively, the person must be a citizen of that country.

Switzerland – Laws and Loopholes

In Switzerland, assisted suicide is allowed by law as long as the person providing the assistance has no selfish motive. Importantly, the person receiving the assistance does not need to be a Swiss citizen. Given that voluntary euthanasia remains illegal in Switzerland, it is interesting that Swiss law has allowed assisted suicide since the 1940s.

In Switzerland, the penal code states that 'a person who, for selfish motives, persuades or assists another person to commit suicide will be punished with imprisonment up to five years.' People other than the 'selfish', commit no crime in assisting others to suicide.

It is not surprising, then, to find that Switzerland harbours several right to die organizations each of which have their own memberships and differing *modus operandi.*

Such groups include the little-known Exit – The Swiss Society for Humane Dying and the much more well known, Dignitas. Dignitas is the main organization to accept foreigners as clients.

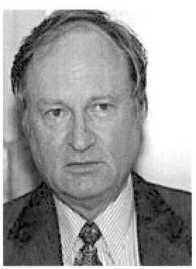

Fig 17.1: Dignitas Director, Ludwig Minelli

Dignitas

Dignitas was established by Ludwig Minelli in 1998 as a Swiss, non-profit organization.

Based in Zurich, Dignitas aims to provide its members with the option of a dignified death. Recognizing the limitations of organizations such as Exit Deutsche Schweiz, which only provide their services to Swiss nationals, Minelli has created a service that caters for an increasing demand around the world.

Dignitas' guidelines state that they assist people who have been diagnosed with a terminal illness, an incurable disease, or who are in a medically hopeless state. Such people may have intolerable pain or an unreasonable handicap. A person does not need to have a terminal illness to be accepted as a client by Dignitas.

Interestingly, Minelli has recently gone further suggesting that people with mental illness should not be automatically excluded from the Dignitas service as their suffering is real and deserves to be addressed as such.

A Word of Warning

While the theory of allowing a dementia sufferer to decide on his or her own suicide is one thing, the reality of doing this is quite different. Suicide by the mentally ill, not simply those affected by diseases such as Alzheimer's, is an area fraught with danger. There is no better example of what can go wrong than the 2008 case of Sydney Exit members, Shirley Justins and Caren Jenning (see Ch 18)

Dignitas does reject a client on the basis of a lack of capacity, that person and their family need to be very careful about alternative strategies.

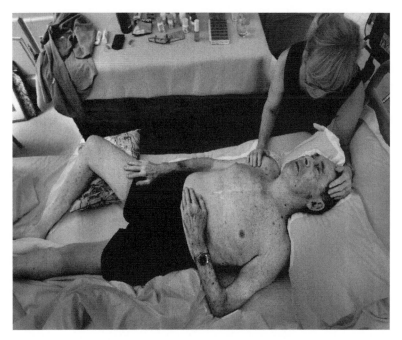

Fig 17.2: Dr Elliott, with Multiple Myeloma

The Dignitas Process

As those who have used the Dignitas service have discovered, nothing happens quickly. The Swiss are, rightly, very particular. This is why it is best to approach Dignitas well ahead of the date of a perceived need. The application process for Dignitas can be lengthy and drawn out.

The first step to using the Dignitas service is to join the organization. For a one-off joining fee of Euros 50 and a yearly membership fee of Euros 25, a person can become a member. From there the person can choose to apply to make use of the service at some time in the future, when/ if the need should arise.

You can join Dignitas by writing to them, emailing or phoning (contact details are given at the end of this Chapter). While a proficiency in German is not mandatory on the telephone, it will help when dealing with more complex questions. The Dignitas phone reception does have an English language option, but this can lead to an answering machine, depending on the time of day you call.

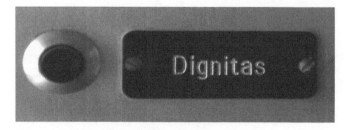

Fig 17.3: The Dignitas Doorbell

To make an application to Dignitas, there is a formidable list of documents required. To be considered by Dignitas, you must have had your illness fully investigated, diagnosed and recorded and an official medical case history compiled in your home country. Documents which may be required by Dignitas upon application include:

- Birth certificate (issued in past 6 months)
- Passport
- Marriage certificate (issued in past 6 months)
- Medical records (tests and results)
- Medical specialist reports
- General Practitioner medical reports
- Current local government rates notice (to prove place of residency)
- Current drivers license
- Statements from family members (children, grandchildren)

To apply to use the Dignitas service, a client needs to complete the application form and forward this, along with copies/ and originals to the Dignitas office in Zurich.

Note – Swiss authorities insist that at least some of these documents are certified extracts, and some may need to be witnessed by a Justice of the Peace or Public Notary. Others may need to have been issued within the last 6 months. Be prepared to do a fair bit of running around to gather the paperwork together.

Upon receipt of this application form, Dignitas reviews each applicant's situation. If deemed suitable, a provisional letter of acceptance will be mailed to the client (called the 'green light'). It is at this point, plans for travel to Zurich can be made.

Upon Arrival in Zurich

Upon arrival in Zurich, the client contacts Dignitas. An appointment is then made with one of a number of consulting physicians who work in conjunction with the organization. These medical doctors are independent of Dignitas and work from their own rooms.

There is a detailed meeting with the consulting doctor and the medical records are re-examined (also by a second doctor). If relatives or loved ones have accompanied the client to Dignitas, the doctor may wish to interview these family members and/ or friends as well. Don't be surprised if you are interviewed together, then individually, then together again.

Once the medical consultation has taken place and if the doctor is satisfied, a prescription for pentobarbital will be written. The drug is not handed over to the client at the time of the consultation with the doctor. Rather, approval at this stage means that the final appointment – the time when the death can take place – is then able to be made. The doctor's approval means that the drug will be available for consumption by the client at the Dignitas house on the chosen day.

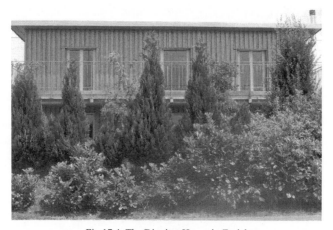

Fig 17.4: The Dignitas House in Zurich

The Final Appointment

The final appointment is held at the Dignitas house in an outer suburb of Zurich. This appointment can take place quite quickly after the medical review, sometimes the following day. Two Dignitas staff will be present.

A third member of the Dignitas team may arrive during the appointment and deliver the drugs that will be used.

The Drugs

As is the case in all places (Netherlands, Belgium, Oregon) where assisted suicide or voluntary euthanasia is legal, the drug that is used at Dignitas is pentobarbital sodium (Nembutal). A prescription will have been written out for this drug by the consulting doctor who saw the client. The prescription would have been filled on your behalf by Dignitas staff.

It is the Dignitas staff who bring the Nembutal to the house for the final appointment. At the appointment, staff dissolve the pentobarbital sodium powder in water to form a drink. This is done when the person indicates that it is their wish to go ahead with their death.

The Pentobarbital used by Dignitas is the soluble sodium salt and 15gm are dissolved in ~50ml of water just before use. The concentration of Nembutal in the liquid consumed is 300mg/ml. The amount consumed is ~50 mls which is no more than a few mouthfuls. Note: This dose differs significantly in concentration from the sterile veterinary anaesthetic Nembutal. Anaesthetic Nembutal has a concentration of 60mg/ml, about 5x weaker than that used by Dignitas.

Dying at Dignitas

Once the client and their family and friends arrive at the Dignitas house for the final appointment, a few further tasks must be attended to. Firstly, additional legal paperwork must be completed concerning informed consent, power of attorney and forms to release the body. This final hurdle clears the way for the death to take place.

At this time, the client reads, approves and once more signs papers indicating that they know what they are about to do and indicating that they are acting of their own free will. Their signature is witnessed by those present. Following the paperwork, the Dignitas staff explain that the person can opt out of the process at any time. The client is asked if they'd prefer to stay seated around the table or if they'd like to lie down. Either way, it is the client who determines what happens and how it happens.

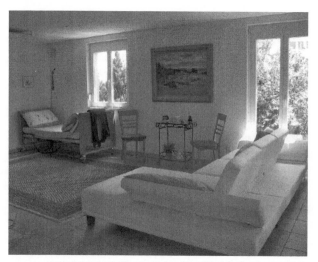

Fig 17.5: One of two rooms at the Dignitas House

The Dignitas rooms are bright, airy welcoming rooms. They are decorated in warm colours. There is a coffee machine and CD player for those who wish to have music. And in case you forget to bring your own music, there is even a Dignitas CD compilation of well known relaxing popular music, in case you feel that music might be a valuable last minute addition.

If the client wishes to go ahead, the staff then set up a video recorder on a tripod in the corner of the room. All proceedings from this point on will be recorded. This is done to provide evidence about the death if questions are asked as to its voluntary nature. After the death, the police may view the tape to ensure that no pressure or coercion took place. With the camera rolling the client is then given access to the first of two drugs. The first drug is an anti-emetic (anti-vomiting drug) and is taken in the form of a small drink. The drug provided is metoclopramide (see Chapter 8). This drug is taken as a stat dose.

The Dignitas staff place the glass on the table and the client can reach for the glass and take the drug if they wish. After this drug is swallowed, a half an hour is needed for it to take effect before proceeding. This time can be very stressful and the Dignitas staff are skilled in providing a calm environment for the client and others who may be present.

When the time has passed, the client is then given access to the Nembutal. Once again, the Dignitas staff ask if the client wishes to proceed, reminding them that they can still opt out or change their mind. If the client wants to proceed, the staff place the small glass of the pentobarbital sodium solution on the table.

In January 2007, the authors accompanied US-born, Sydney doctor, John Elliott, to the Dignitas clinic. Dying of multiple myeloma (a cancer of the bone marrow), this 79-year old man's last weeks had been a nightmare and he wanted release from his suffering.

John was very keen to find peace. When presented with the glass of Nembutal, he reached for it quickly. However, John had a problem with gastric reflux, a condition associated with the palliative radiation therapy he had undergone some weeks earlier.

Afraid that he would vomit, John needed some reassurance and was pleased when he was able to consume the 50ml drink with little difficulty. Prepared for a bitter after-taste, he finished the Nembutal, saying 'that didn't taste too bad.'

Because John's favourite drink was cognac, everyone shared his final moments with a toast. Not only did the cognac take away the drug's after-taste, it made the Nembutal work faster.

We clinked glasses and, while his wife Angelika held him, John nodded peacefully off to sleep. John Elliott died within the hour. John's journey has been captured in a short film called 'Flight to Zurich.' See: *http://www.youtube.com/watch?v=1j4c6aVFfUk*

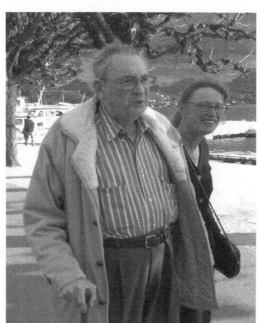

Fig 17.6: Dr John Elliott and his wife Angelika in Switzerland shortly before his death

After it's Over

After about an hour, one of the Dignitas staff members performed several simple tests to confirm death. Once this was established, the staff called the police who arrived with a medical doctor and an officer from the Coroner's department. The funeral home was also contacted at this time. In all deaths, those present are asked to leave the room while the doctor examines the body, The police may view the video tape of the death and interview those present about the nature of the death. Was the death peaceful? Was it voluntary? Did it go according to the person's wishes?

Once all questions are answered and the officials are comfortable, the family and friends of the deceased person can leave. The body is then removed to the funeral home, in preparation for either cremation or transportation back to the person's country of origin.

Dignitas and the Swiss Law

While the statistics tend to vary, Dignitas staff confirm that around 300 people use their assisted suicide service each year. Well over half of these people are from countries other than Switzerland.

Although there have been a handful of situations where a client's family has become disgruntled with Dignitas (these cases have been reported at length in the international media), most people are grateful to Ludwig Minelli and his compassionate team of workers who make this choice in dignified dying possible.

If you are thinking about using the Dignitas service, there are several points to note. Firstly, it is important to understand that Dignitas does not provide voluntary euthanasia. Swiss law does not allow a doctor to administer a lethal injection to a client. The client must be able to act for themselves and consume the lethal drug unassisted. This means that unless a person is able move their arms to lift the glass to their lips, or suck on a straw, or swallow, or empty the drug into their own stomach 'peg', then Dignitas is not the service for them.

Remember, at Dignitas there is no doctor present at the death. Once a person has been accepted by Dignitas, this is very much a DIY model of operation. Interestingly, Dignitas Founder - Ludwig Minelli - has a professional background in law not medicine. Dignitas provides as de-medicalised a model of dying as Swiss law will allow.

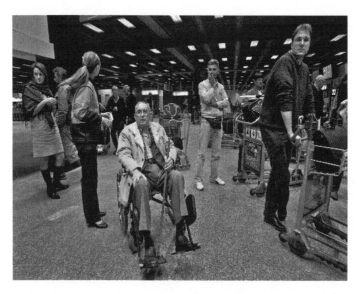

Fig 17.7: John Elliott on arrival at Zurich Airport

Finally, Dignitas is unique in that it represents the only legal option for dignified dying for people living outside of jurisdictions where voluntary euthanasia and assisted suicide are legal. In Exit's opinion the popularity of the service is likely to continue, although the distance those suffering must travel ensures that Dignitas will never be first choice for those in the southern hemisphere.

Dignitas' Future

In March 2011, the good people of the Canton of Zurich went to referendum to decide if the Dignitas service should be able to continue accepting foreigners as clients.

Despite grave fears, the population voted overwhelmingly (78%) to maintain the status quo allowing foreigners access to Switzerland's assisted suicide services.

Media reports about this positive development can be found at:
http://www.bbc.co.uk/news/world-europe-13405376
http://bit.ly/lcpjpb

Dignitas Costs

At the current time, the Dignitas organization charges a one-off joining fee of approximately Euros 50 and an annual member contribution of at least Euros 25. The current cost of the Dignitas service starts at around ten thousand euro.

Dignitas Contact Details

Address:
PO Box 9, CH 8127
Forch, Switzerland

Telephone: 0011 41 44 980 44 59
Fax: 0011 41 44 980 14 21
Email: dignitas@dignitas.ch
Website: http://www.dignitas.ch

18

After it's Over

Introduction

For those left behind, the period immediately following the death of a loved one can be an intensely sad and stressful time. An elected death - a rational suicide - can present an additional and unique set of circumstances.

On the one hand, family and friends may be enormously relieved that their loved one was able to die peacefully and with dignity. On the other hand, there may be feelings of resentment, even anger that the person they loved has chosen to leave them. While it is one thing to know that a person you love is about to die by their own hand, it is another to be able to predict how this will make you feel.

There will also be a number of practical issues that those left behind have to confront. In the case of a well planned death, some of these will have been discussed before the death. For example, will anyone be responsible for clearing away any used equipment from the scene of death? And what about a suicide note? Who will keep hold of it, should one be required?

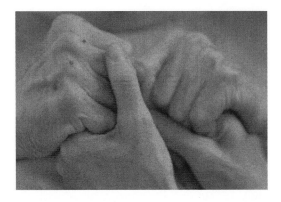

Then there is the issue of having the death certificate signed, and whether or not an autopsy will be conducted. Will there will be a coronial investigation? Many of these issues can be anticipated and prepared for. In this Chapter we use the real life example of Australian former Qantas pilot Graeme Wylie to illustrate what not to do when someone decides to take their own life. We point identify some of the factors which will contribute towards a well planned death.

Background to Graeme Wylie

In March 2006 Graeme Wylie died drinking a lethal dose of veterinary Nembutal that his friend of over 30 years, Caren Jenning, had brought back for him from Mexico. While the plan and Caren's motive for helping her old friend were straight forward, Graeme Wylie's death was always going to be complicated. In June 2008, Graeme Wylie's partner of 18 years Shirley Justins, together with Caren, was found guilty of his manslaughter and accessory to manslaughter respectively.

Graeme Wylie was suffering from dementia, anything from 'mild to moderate' to 'moderate to severe' depending on which doctor carried out the assessment. In the court case that followed his death, Graeme Wylie was deemed not to have had the 'capacity' to know what he was doing by drinking the Nembutal. Graeme did not, therefore, take his own life. Rather the court found he was 'killed' by Shirley and Caren.

The first issue that a person considering taking their own life should consider is whether they have the capacity to make the decision? While the Wylie case is an extreme example, to keep loved ones safe the question should be asked. Another sensible step is to pen a suicide note in one's own hand.

The Suicide Note

If Graeme Wylie had written, signed and dated a suicide note stating that his actions were entirely his own, that he understood the consequences of what he was about to do and gave the reasons for dying, Shirley and Caren would have been much less likely to have found themselves in front of a judge and jury.

The law around suicide and assisted-suicide is grey. Those left behind by a death are almost always at risk of some form of inquisition from authorities. Writing a note and storing it in a safe place or with a trusted friend makes a good deal of sense. In a well-planned death, a doctor should simply sign the death certificate, believing that the death is natural and a result of the underlying disease. In cases like these, the suicide note will never be needed.

If, however, like Graeme Wylie, the doctor refuses to sign the death certificate, the coroner is contacted and an autopsy is arranged, then this is the time for the signed suicide note to be 'found'. In this scenario, the suicide note will provide a very useful safeguard if loved ones find themselves implicated in the death. If on the other hand, the person taking their life does not care that their death be a known suicide, the note can be left alongside their body.

The Process of a Death

If a death takes place outside of a hospital, hospice or other medical institution (eg. at home), it is normal practice upon 'discovering' the death, that a doctor be called. Upon arriving at the house, the doctor will then have two options.

If the death looks to be natural, and the patient has been seen by the doctor in the past two months, the doctor will certify death and sign the death certificate citing the person's underlying disease as the cause of death. There will be no red tape. The body will be released, and funeral arrangements can be made.

If, on the other hand, the doctor suspects that the death is *not* natural (eg. if the death is possibly a suicide or if the cause of death is unclear) the doctor can certify death, but will not sign the death certificate. In this case the doctor will call the coroner's office and the police will be involved. Those close to the deceased may be required to be interviewed by the police about their relationship with the deceased, and about their possible role in the person's death.

If the deceased was known to be seriously ill and if that person has made an effort to choose a method that leaves no obvious physical signs, or if the person and/or friends and family have ensured that any evidence of suicide is removed from the scene, the doctor will likely certify death *and* sign the death certificate.

While Graeme Wylie had dementia, he had no other underlying physical illness that could have explained his cause of death. He was 71 years of age and physically fit when he died. His death was, therefore, immediately suspicious. Knowing this in advance, Caren and Shirley attempted to suggest that the cause of his death was down to the medication he was taking, a drug called Aricept. They did this by showing the attending police an article from the *New York Times*. The article highlighted a link between Aricept and heart attack in dementia patients. The police did not buy their story. At autopsy, Graeme Wylie's body was found to contain lethal levels of pentobarbital (Nembutal).

When attending a death, police are usually very sensitive and respectful. However, they are there to do a job and this may involve the questioning of those who were in the house at the time. The police may also look at the degree of incapacitation of the person who has died. If an obvious suicide they will note whether or not the method used could have been carried out solely by the individual. Any need for help or assistance to suicide is evidence of a crime.

If there is any doubt, the questioning of those left behind may intensify. The issue of whether anyone was present when the suicide took place may also arise. In this situation, there is no guarantee that legal action will not be taken against a person who admits to simply being present, even if they say they did nothing to assist.

Note: Police do not attend all deaths. They will only attend deaths that are suspicious. In recent months, Exit has learned of at least two members who have died whose families have then been quizzed by the authorities. The reason? They were members of Exit. If this happens to you, say nothing on or off the record and never submit to a policy interview unless you have an attorney present. Seek legal advice immediately.

Cleaning Away

There are several practical steps that can be taken to increase the likelihood that a death will be seen as 'natural' (if that is what the deceased person wished). The first of these is the act of cleaning up after a death.

Given that the deaths that we are talking about are peaceful and dignified, the act of cleaning up generally involves the removal of equipment such as an Exit Bag or empty drug packets from the death scene. In some situations, this can be done well ahead of time. Many people ending their lives clean away themselves. They remove drug-packaging, and rinse glasses after a lethal drug has been consumed. If this is done, the attending doctor will be more likely to assume that the cause of death is the underlying disease.

However, if the person who has died was not known to be suffering from a life threatening illness, the act of cleaning away may cause more problems. In the case of Graeme Wylie, because there was no illness (other than dementia), the fact that there was no obvious cause of death only served to heighten the mystery of how he died?

If Graeme Wylie had written a note and left the bottle of Nembutal alongside him, instead of the bottle being removed by his wife so it would never be found, the police would have known immediately that his death was a suicide.

If a person ends their life using an Exit Bag, then the cleaning away will involve the removal of the bag from the person's head along with the helium cylinder and tubing. Occasionally at Helium deaths the bag, gas control fitting and tubing are all that is removed. If the black and white plastic nozzle that came with the balloon kit is re-attached, the cylinder re-boxed and re-stored in the cupboard, it is unlikely the cylinder will be linked to the death.

For a death to appear normal, there must be no evidence of equipment that could have been used in the suicide. While some people might not care whether their death is listed as 'suicide' or 'natural', the legal risk to others will be higher if it is known a suicide has taken place.

Cleaning Away and the Law

While it can be an offence to interfere with the 'circumstances of a death'/ 'interfere with a corpse' etc, in the scheme of things it is not a particularly serious one. For example, removing an Exit bag from a loved one's head once they have died is a very different matter to helping that same person put the bag on their head. It is clearly assisting a suicide to help a person position a bag on their head. In most western countries, assisting a suicide is a serious crime.

If, by chance, the authorities do learn that some 'cleaning-up' has taken place, family and friends often explain their actions by saying that they were protecting the family's reputation. They say it would be a blemish on the person's good name if their suicide were ever to be made public. Generally speaking, the act of 'cleaning away' is unlikely to attract anything more than a legal slap on the wrist.

Death Certificates

Upon arriving at the scene, the attending family doctor will perform two tasks. Firstly, they will confirm death. They will do this by carrying out a number of simple tests to establish that the person is indeed dead, not simply in a catatonic or comatose state. Having confirmed death, the next issue is the signing of the death certificate. There are a number of requirements that must be satisfied before this can be done. Two are of particular interest.

1. The doctor must know the patient. Usually there is the requirement that the doctor has seen the patient in a professional capacity - not just to say hello at the golf club - in the past two months (the time period varies depending on the jurisdiction).
2. The doctor must be satisfied that the death is natural.

The requirement that the patient be known to the doctor can sometimes cause difficulty. Often, very sick people have little contact with the medical profession. This means that finding a doctor who could even sign the certificate can be a problem. It may therefore be wise to call your doctor for a visit prior to the planned death, complaining of a developing fever or breathlessness, perhaps some pain on deep inspiration.

When the doctor is then called back some days later, it would reasonable for them to assume a natural death involving pneumonia.

Some people worry a great deal about the way their death will be recorded on their death certificate. They fear being known as someone who 'committed suicide.' Others have no preference, saying 'who cares what they write, I'll be dead anyway?'

If a person who is about to die from a terminal disease takes their own life, the death will be recorded as 'suicide.' If that person does not want 'suicide' recorded on the death certificate, they will need to take steps to disguise the truth. A method of death that leaves no obvious signs is of course the only logical course.

Dying without Trace

Most drugs used to end life leave no obvious identifying signs. Death from sterile veterinary Nembutal is one example. The person will appear as if they succumbed to their cancer or heart disease. However, there is also a dyed form of the drug, Pentobarbital (see Chapter 13). If Lethobarb (the dyed form) is consumed, the person's lips will be stained green; hence the name the 'green dream'. Green lips are a dead giveaway (pardon the pun) to a death that is not natural. And remember, if an autopsy is performed, the pentobarbital will be discovered. Questions about its source will inevitably be asked. This is true of any death brought about by a consumed drug, or an inhaled poison like carbon monoxide.

The *only method* that leaves no trace, even at autopsy, is the Exit Bag with nitrogen (a hypoxic death with helium will be detectable at autopsy). For the death to be recorded as natural, however, the bag, flow control fitting, tubing and the helium canister would need to be removed. It can be useful if a family member or friend can 'discover' the body in the morning. This person will then be in a position to call the family doctor and remind the doctor of the underlying illness. One can also claim that everyone in the house was asleep during the evening when the death took place.

Autopsies

If there is any doubt about the cause of death, the doctor will contact the coroner and an autopsy may be arranged. An autopsy involves the dissection of the body by a pathologist, the visual and microscopic inspection of organs, and the biochemical testing of body fluids, stomach contents etc.

At autopsy, the existence of any drugs (and alcohol) in the body will be discovered. If the drug is uncommon or difficult to obtain, questions will be asked about whether or not assistance was provided in obtaining, preparing or administering the substance.

Although permission for an autopsy will be sought, and next of kin have the right to refuse, it is as well to remember that refusal can generally be overridden (depending upon the jurisdiction). Autopsies are generally only sought if there is a legal or medical mystery associated with the death; that is, if there is uncertainty about how or why the person died. In these situations, especially if there is the possibility of a criminal act (eg. assistance), the decision will be made irrespective of family wishes.

In cases where the death is clearly a suicide, an autopsy will not necessarily be performed. Autopsies are expensive and only undertaken if a benefit can be established. They are also undertaken for political reasons. When Caren Jenning took her own life in September 2008, a month before she was due to be sentenced for the manslaughter of Graeme Wylie, she left a suicide note and the bottle of Nembutal by her bed. Nevertheless an autopsy was still performed. Her reputation preceded her, even in death.

Even though autopsies are by no means routine, and their use is becoming less frequent, they can never be ruled out (O'Connor, 2004). Still, in the case of a seriously ill person who takes an overdose of prescription propoxyphene they have had prescribed, *and* leaves the empty packets by the bed, *and* a suicide note, there is little likelihood of an autopsy being performed. Remember the only method which will not be discovered at autopsy is a hypoxic death using Nitrogen (see Chapter 5 for full details).

Grief Counselling

The suicide of a seriously ill person will evoke mixed reactions in those close to that person. The broader community's reaction may also be mixed. While most people support the concept of rational suicide there is still a significant minority who do not. It cannot be assumed that there will always be sympathy for those left behind so be careful.

In many circumstances where a person has died of their own hand, counselling may be of assistance for those left behind. The ability to talk things through can be therapeutic and can go a long way towards easing the inevitable grief and despair.

Private counsellors list their services in most countries' telephone directories and of course online. Community health centres also commonly offer counselling as part of their range of health services. There are also often community telephone help lines.

Telling Your Story Publicly

Many suffering people who choose to end their life, resent the fact that they have to act like criminals in order to die with dignity. Some choose to travel overseas to acquire prohibited drugs. Others lie to their doctors and deceive those they love. Many are acutely conscious that in most western jurisdictions, this is an unsatisfactory situation. All of us want change for the better.

For all these reasons, some people want their deaths to mean something. Telling their story in the media is one way they believe (and Exit agrees) to push the debate forward.

If you are a person who wants to contribute to public debate and encourage our legislators to act, there are several options available. As a rule of thumb, most media are keen on personal stories that involve suffering and heroism. There are however drawbacks to such actions and they can be significant.

If the personal story of a forthcoming death is made public, there can be considerable scrutiny of the individual and possible frustration of their plans. The death of Australian grandmother, Nancy Crick, was an example of this. Nancy went public with her plans to die well before the night she eventually drank her Nembutal with 21 friends and family present. While telling her story forced key establishment figures to engage with the issue of a person's right to choose when and how they die, the exact time and place of her suicide turned into a bit of a media circus. Nevertheless she died peacefully, sipping on Baileys and smoking her last cigarette.

Over the years, Exit has found an alternative approach is for the person to record their story, or film an interview, with the provision that it be published only after their death. This was the case with 31-year-old Angelique Flowers. Angelique's Internet plea to the Australian Prime Minister was front page news in the Melbourne broadsheet *The Age*. And, as discussed in Chapter 1 of this *Handbook*, her video diary remains available on *YouTube* to this day. While such statements can be very powerful, the fact that when they are only made known after the person has died can limit on-going media interest.

It is also important to remember that tapes and records can be subpoenaed and possibly used as evidence. It was the airing on *60 Minutes* of a video tape of Dr Kevorkian assisting his patient, Thomas Youk, that saw Kevorkian spend nearly a decade in prison.

A third possible way to tell your story publicly is for your family and those closest to you to tell your story after you have gone. This of course is a very safe option. Without the imagery and direct quotes of the person, however, there will be much less media interest and impact. All that said, getting people's stories out to the broader public domain is an essential part of initiating political change.

Concluding Comments

The Peaceful Pill Handbook (PPH) was first published in 2006. Since this time the book has been regularly updated to include new and changed information. This is essential to keep up with the debate about end of life choices.

In 2008, the fully-online *Peaceful Pill eHandbook (PPeH)* was released. The online format of the *eHandbook* has allowed updating when and as it is required. At the current time, the *eHandbook* is updated six times each year.

The online *eHandbook* also contains over 50 pieces of video, providing hands-on instruction and critical detail on a diverse range of issues.

For readers of the *PPH*, Exit is pleased to continue to offer a cash-back arrangement should purchasers upgrade to an online subscription to the *PPeH*.

Both books are made available in the philosophical belief that knowledge is empowering. With the academic literature playing catch-up, Exit remains acutely aware that having an end-of-life plan makes one live a longer and happier life. Far from pushing people towards suicide, establishing one's options helps people stop worrying, and get on with living better. For those with terminal illness, being back in control can be pretty satisfying given the adversity that often circles about.

Freedom shouldn't take this much effort. But for the time being it does. Exit appreciates reader feedback on the facts and the feelings that come with reading our books.

Index

Exit RP Test

	Hanging	Detergent	Monoxide	Morphine	Endep	Doloxene	Cyanide	Inert Gas	Nembutal
Reliable (10)	10	10	8	4	9	9	10	8	10
Peaceful (10)	0	2	7	10	7	7	5	7	10
Available (5)	5	5	3	3	3	4	2	5	2
Preparation (5)	2	4	1	5	3	3	5	1	5
Undetectable (5)	0	0	1	2	3	3	3	5*	4
Speed (5)	1	5	5	2	2	2	5	5	4
Safety (5)	5	0	1	5	5	5	3	5	5
Storage (5)	5	4	4	3	3	3	5	5	4
TOTAL (50)	28	30	31	34	35	36	38	41	44
%	56%	60%	62%	68%	70%	72%	76%	82%	88%
Rating	9	8	7	6	5	4	3	2	1

* Nitrogen only

References

Australian Bureau of Statistics (2000) *Suicide Trends, Australia, 1921-1998*. Cat. No. 3309.0, Canberra, ABS.

Australian Veterinary Association (2006) 'AVA rejects Nitschke advice as unethical' Media Release 24 July, 2006.

Batlle, J. C. (2003) 'Legal status of physician-assisted suicide', *JAMA*, Vol. 289, No. 17, p. 2279-81.

Commonwealth of Australia (2005) Criminal Code Amendment (Suicide Related Material Offences) Act 2005 NO. 92 at: *http://www.austlii.edu.au/au/legis/cth/num_act/ccarmoa2005n922005479/*

Drug Misuse and Trafficking Act 1985 (NSW) at: *http://www.austlii.edu.au/au/legis/nsw/consol_act/dmata1985256/index.html*

Furniss, B., Hannaford, A. Smith, P. W. G. & A. Tatchell (1989) *Vogels's Textbook of Practical Organic Chemistry,* Harlow, Prentice Hall.

Hancock, D. (2005) 'Deaths Cocktail', *The Bulletin*, 8 Nov at: *http://www.exitinternational.net/documents/exit45.pdf*

Humphry, D. (1996) *Final Exit*. New York, Dell, p. 30.

Liebermann, L. (2003) *Leaving You – The Cultural Meaning of Suicide*. Chicago, Ivan R. Dee.

Mendelson, W. B. (1980) *The Use and Misuse of Sleeping Pills - a Clinical Guide*, New York, Plenum Medical Book Company.

References

National Prescribing Centre (2006) 'The withdrawal of co-proxamol: alternative analgesics for mild to moderate pain' *MeReC Bulletin*, Vol. 16, No. 4.

Nitschke, P. & Stewart, F. (2005) *Killing Me Softly: VE and the Road to the Peaceful Pill*. Melbourne, Penguin.

O'Connor, A. (2004) 'Deaths go unexamined and the living pay the price', *New York Times*, 2 March.

Public Citizen (2006) 'Petition to the FDA to ban all pro-poxyphene (Darvon) products at: *http://www.citizen.org/publications/release.cfm?ID=7420*

Routley, V. & Ozanne-Smith, J. (1998) 'The impact of catalytic converters on motor vehicle exhaust gas suicides', *Medical Journal of Australia*. Vol. 168, p. 65-67.

Ryan, C. J. (1996) 'Depression, decisions and the desire to die', *Medical Journal of Australia*, Vol. 165, p. 411.

Shanahan, D. (2001) 'Mail order suicide kit', *The Australian*. 20 August.

Solomons, T. W. B. & Fryhle, C. B. (2004) *Organic Chemistry* (8th ed.), New Jersey, John Wiley & Sons.

Stone, G. (2001) *Suicide and Attempted Suicide: Methods and Consequences*, New York, Carroll and Graf.

Veterinary Surgeons Board of the ACT (2003) *Newsletter* June 2003

About Philip Nitschke

Dr Philip Nitschke PhD, MBBS, BSc (Hons) is a leading authority on Voluntary Euthanasia and Assisted Suicide. As the first doctor in the world to administer a legal, lethal, voluntary injection under Australia's short-lived *Rights of the Terminally Ill Act*, Philip has experienced all sides of the end-of-life choices debate.

A graduate of Sydney University Medical School, Philip is the Founder and Director of Exit International, an organisation at the forefront of this debate. With his co-author Fiona Stewart he is also author of *Killing Me Softly: Voluntary Euthanasia and the Road to the Peaceful Pill* (Penguin 2005, republished Exit US 2011). His autobiography *Damned If I Do* (with Peter Corris) was published by Melbourne University Press in 2013.

In 1997, Philip was awarded the Rainier Foundation Humanitarian Award in the US and was Australian Northern Territorian of the Year. In 1998, Philip was Australian Humanist of the Year and New Zealand Humanist of the year in 2001. He has been nominated for Australian of the Year eight times.

About Fiona Stewart

Dr Fiona Stewart PhD, MPolLaw, GradDip PubPol, BA is a public health sociologist. Fiona has held various positions within and outside the academy including as a journalist, columnist, dot-com founder and media strategist. She is currently completing a post-graduate law degree.

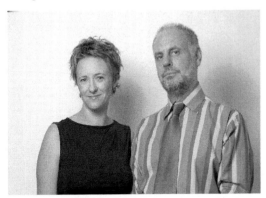

Fiona Stewart & Philip Nitschke

The Peaceful Pill Forums

Members of Exit have free access (on approval) to
the *Peaceful Pill* Discussion Forums at:
www.peacefulpillforums.com

This is an online space where folk can ask
questions about issues covered in the
eHandbook and benefit from the comments, advice
and experience of experts, other subscribers
and Exit members.

Note: Purchasers of the Print edition *Peaceful Pill
Handbook* are entitled to a US$10 cashback should
they elect to upgrade to a subscription to the online
Peaceful Pill eHandbook. This payment is made
after purchase by check.

Join Exit International

exit

Membership of Exit Internationa provides:

* Exit meetings & workshops (free for members)
* Exit R&D (barbiturate testing & analysis, inert gas strategies - helium/ nitrogen)
* Local Chapters
* Peaceful Pill Online Forums (free & exclusive for members)
* Private Visits
* Exit Newsletter *Deliverance*
* Exit Supporter lapel badge & card

First Name..................................Last Name..

Address...

....Postcode.............
.
Email...Date of Birth......................................

Phone...Occupation...

Exit Membership is A$100 ($110 if in Australia inc $10 gst)
(Life Membership is granted for gifts of $1000 or more)

Visa ☐   Mastercard ☐   Cash/Money Order ☐   Check ☐

Credit Card No................................Name on Card............................

Expiry date ..../.................Signature..

Exit International USA
PO Box 4250
Bellingham WA 98227
USA

Ph (+1) 360-347-1810
Fax (+1) 360-844-1501

contact@exitinternational.net
www.exitinernational.net
www.peacefulpill.com